CPEN®
Study Guide
2024

Pamela D. Bartley, BSN, RN, CEN, TCRN, CCRN-K, CFRN, CPEN

I have 40 years of experience as an emergency/critical care nurse and educator. My passion is assisting nurses achieve their certification goals. Thank you for selecting me as your certification mentor and for supporting a nurse-owned small business.

Follow **www.pdbnurseeducationllc.com** for blog posts.

Email me at pbartleysc@gmail.com if you have any questions.

PDB Nurse Education, LLC
CPEN Study Tips (12 Step-by-Step Guide)

1. Thank you for allowing me to be your certification mentor! This is a commitment, but we can and WILL DO IT. Email me at **pbartleysc@gmail.com** if you have questions (do not message me please). Download the exam blueprint at www.BCEN.org.
2. Check out **"Don't Forget the Bubbles"** and **"PedEMMorsels"** websites for great resources.
3. **Register for the CPEN exam soon**, it makes it "real", and you will actively study. Do not tell anyone when your test date is, that just adds more pressure. You have **90 days to take the exam once you register**, but please do not schedule the exam for day 90, because something may go wrong. Check www.BCEN.org for exam information.
4. **Schedule your exam at the best time of day for you, morning, or afternoon.** When are you most alert – am or pm? Schedule your test for that time of day.
5. The CEN exam is **175 questions, and you have 180 minutes** to complete. All questions are multiple-choice, not "all of the above" or "select all that apply". You **must score 110/150 that are graded, 73% correct to pass.**
6. Yes, the **CPEN 2022 pass rate was 55%**, but if you follow my advice, you have a much higher chance of passing the exam. No, my pass rate is not 100%.
7. **Twenty-five questions on the exam do not count**, BCEN is testing emergency nursing knowledge of some concepts. The 25 questions can be anywhere on exam, just make the best educated choice.
8. The CPEN exam has **6 sections**, study one section per week or two after you take ENPC and PALS.
9. Prepare a dedicated study space, just like students in virtual school.
10. Review **"PALS Review" and "Physiology Review"** creating flashcards of content you do not fully comprehend. Study the **175 "Sample Questions"** until you fully understand them. Ensure you make 75% on the **"CPEN Posttest"** The **100 "Critical Thinking**" questions will safeguard that you have a handle on the content.
11. **Study during your peak brain time** and consider playing instrumental music while you study to stimulate your brain. Study in 30-45-minute intervals, then exercise before continuing.
12. What **study strategy** works best for you?
    a. Talk to a nurse who recently passed the CPEN exam and ask for suggestions. This exam has evolved over the last 5 years, focusing more on prioritization and critical thinking, not memorization. Review **ESI 5th edition and ENPC 6th edition** to help with prioritization questions.
    b. I strongly suggest you have a study buddy to keep you accountable.
    c. Develop **flash cards** of concepts you do not fully understand, **not everything**. Take the flashcards to work and ask everyone to tell you everything they know about that concept.
    d. **Develop memory aids**, mnemonics, and acronyms for communicable diseases, antidotes, etc.
    e. Take the timed version of the **BCEN's sample 150 questions for $40** if you feel you need additional sample questions.
    f. **Record** yourself explaining **"Key Points"** in your own words and listen while driving or exercising, or before going to bed.
    g. **Explain difficult material** to a co-worker and encourage questions. You know the material when you can teach it to someone else.
    h. You can purchase BCEN **test assurance** vouchers to reduce test anxiety and test through live remote proctoring if you are more testing comfortable at home.

- **PALS Science Update 2020 pg. 9**
    - Target respiratory rate of 20-30 breaths/minute **(1 breath every 2-3 seconds).**
    - Use **cuffed ET tube** to improve accuracy of capnography and decrease risk of aspiration.
    - Consider naloxone (Narcan) in respiratory arrest due to suspected opioid overdose (pinpoint pupils).
    - Fluid bolus in sepsis **10-20 mL/kg**, repeat as needed.
- **Pediatric BLS - Chapter 2, BLS Summary pg. 81**
    - Check for responsiveness, shout for help, activate EMS. Assess for breathing and pulse, taking no more than 10 seconds. Feel for a brachial pulse in infant, and a carotid or femoral pulse in the child.
    - If the heart rate is < 60/minute with signs of poor perfusion, start CPR. If heart rate is > 60/minute, continue rescue breathing and check the pulse every 2 minutes. If you are alone and witness collapse, activate EMS. **If not a sudden arrest, activate EMS after 2 minutes of CPR.**
    - Infant compressions – 2-finger or 2 thumb-encircling hands technique. Child compressions – 1 or 2 hands. The compression rate is 100-120/minute. Compression-to-ventilation rate for single rescuers is 30:2. **If 2 rescuers are present, use a rate of 15:2 in infants and children**. Allow complete chest recoil. AED– Child pads if available if < age 8. Adult pads if child pads are not available.
- **PALS Systematic Approach - Chapter 4 – Algorithm pg. 38**
    - Pediatric Assessment Triangle (**PAT**) pg. 37 – Across-the-room Assessment of **A**ppearance, Work of **B**reathing, **C**irculation (Color)
        - **A**ppearance – interactivity, muscle tone, cry. **TICLS** – **T**one, **I**nteractiveness, **C**onsolability, **L**ook/gaze, **S**peech/cry.
        - Work of **B**reathing – tripod or sniffing position, nasal flaring, retractions, audible breath sounds (grunting, stridor, wheezing).
        - **C**irculation (Color) – pale, mottled, cyanotic, petechiae, purpura, or obvious bleeding.
    - **Primary Assessment pgs. 44-68, 286-287**
        - **A**irway, **B**reathing, **C**irculation, **D**isability, **E**xposure
        - **A**irway – look, listen, feel, allow position of comfort, or elevate head of bed.
            - **FBAO** – Perform 5 back slaps and 5 chest compressions for under age 1. Abdominal thrusts for 1 year of age and older. Begin CPR if unresponsive.
        - **B**reathing – assess work of breathing and **oxygen saturation** (normal > 94%). Monitor for tachypnea, hyperpnea (deep breathing), bradypnea, or apnea.
            - **Retractions pg. 48 –** subcostal, substernal, intercostal are mild to moderate. Supraclavicular, suprasternal, sternal are severe. Head bobbing seen in respiratory failure. Seesaw respirations seen in neuromuscular weakness.
        - **C**irculation – assess heart rate and rhythm, **central versus peripheral pulses**, capillary refill time (normal is 2 seconds or less), skin color and temperature, blood pressure. Normal urine output is 1.5 to 2 mL/kg/hour in infants and young children, 1 mL/kg/hour in older children and adolescents. **Flash capillary refill and bounding pulses seen in early sepsis**.
        - **D**isability – assess LOC, pupillary response, **blood glucose test**.
            - **AVPU** pg. 60 [**A**lert (15), Response to **V**oice (13), Response to **P**ain (8), **U**nresponsive (6)] GCS equivalents in parentheses. Glasgow Coma Scale **GCS** pgs. 60-61 (mild head injury 13-15, moderate 9-12, severe 3-8)
            - **Hypoglycemia** is blood glucose 45 mg/dL or less in newborn, 60 mg/dL or less in a child. Pg. 63
        - **E**xposure – pg. 63 – assess for evidence of trauma, petechiae and purpura.
    - **Breath sounds pgs. 50-51**
        - **Stridor/Barking – upper airway obstruction**, initially heard on **inspiration**.
        - **Wheezing – lower airway obstruction**, initially heard on **exhalation**.
        - **Grunting** – lung tissue disease, heard on exhalation against a partially closed glottis.
        - Crackles – crackling inspiratory sounds from alveolar fluid.
        - Snoring respirations – indicates an airway obstruction, so **reposition airway**.

- Normal vital signs by age
    - Respiratory rates by age pg. 46, Heart rate by age pg. 53
    - Blood pressure by age pg. 58 **[Hypotension is < 70 + (age in years x 2]**
- Oxygen saturation **< 94% on rom air indicates hypoxemia** pg. 52.
- Pupils pg. 62 – pinpoint in opioid ingestion, **dilated in sympathomimetic** or anticholinergic ingestion, ipsilateral dilated seen in increased ICP and herniation.
- SAMPLE History mnemonic pgs. 64-65 – **S**igns and **S**ymptoms, **A**llergies, **M**edications, **P**ast medical history, **L**ast meal, **E**vents leading to current illness or injury.

- **Recognizing and Managing Cardiac Arrest – Chapter 5**
    - Hypoxic/asphyxia is the **most common cause of pediatric cardiac arrest**.
    - **Sudden cardiac arrest** from cardiomyopathy, Long QT syndrome, myocarditis, drug intoxication, commotio cordis (blow to chest).
    - Recognizing **Cardiac Arrest** pgs. 77-79 Rhythm strips of Asystole, PEA (no pulse), Ventricular fibrillation, Ventricular tachycardia, and Torsades de pointes.
    - Intravenous/**Intraosseous** pgs. 84-85 – any PALS drug can be administered IV or IO. Initiate IO if poor perfusion. Endotracheal medication route – Epinephrine at 10 times the IV/IO dose. Other drugs 2-3 times the IV/IO dose.
    - **Pediatric Cardiac Arrest Medications** pgs. 86-87 - Epinephrine every 3-5 minutes, Amiodarone, Lidocaine, Magnesium sulfate, Atropine, Calcium, Sodium bicarbonate.
    - **Pulseless Cardiac Arrest algorithm** pg. 89 – Focus is CPR and defibrillation, immediately resume compressions after defibrillation.
    - **Defibrillation** pgs. 90-92 – **initial wattage is 2-4 J/kg**, up to 10 J/kg. Use infant pads for < 10 kg or younger than 1 year. "Clear for shock".
    - Cardiac arrest due to **Trauma** pg. 99 – open airway using jaw-thrust, needle decompression for tension pneumothorax, transfuse blood to treat shock, pericardiocentesis for cardiac tamponade, and administer vasopressors for neurogenic shock.
    - Cardiac arrest due to **Drowning** pg. 100 – wipe off chest before defibrillation, restrict spinal motion, suction airway, insert gastric tube, rewarm for severe hypothermia (< 30 degrees C).
    - Cardiac arrest due to **Anaphylaxis** pg. 101 – isotonic fluid boluses and epinephrine.
- **Respiratory Distress/Failure – Chapters 7 & 8**
    - **Recognition of Respiratory Distress/Failure Flowchart pg. 122**
        - **Respiratory distress** – tachypnea, nasal flaring, retractions, pallor, irritability, tripod.
        - Progresses to **Respiratory failure** – bradypnea to apnea, bradycardia, altered LOC (**lethargy),** head bobbing, hypoxia despite oxygenation.
    - **Upper airway obstruction** – FBAO, airway swelling from anaphylaxis, croup, or epiglottitis, abscess. S/S: drooling, stridor on **inspiration**.
        - **Croup** pg. 128 – humidified oxygen, **nebulized epinephrine if stridor at rest,** dexamethasone.
        - **Anaphylaxis** pg. 129 – **IM epinephrine**, repeated as needed, albuterol, methylprednisolone, diphenhydramine, isotonic crystalloids.
    - **Lower airway obstruction – S/S: wheezing** and prolonged expiratory phase.
        - **Bronchiolitis** pg. 131 – suctioning, high-flow oxygen if O_2 sat < 94%, possible albuterol.
        - **Asthma** – pgs. 132-133 – keep O_2 sat > 94% with NRB, high-flow nasal cannula, or NIPPV, **albuterol**, ipratropium bromide, corticosteroids, magnesium sulfate IV infusion.
            - Using a **nebulizer** pg. 159 – add medication, flow at 5-6 L/minute, until no mist. Tell the child, "Take long, slow, deep breaths through your mouth."
            - Using a **metered-dose inhaler (MDI) with a spacer device** pg. 160 – shake the MDI. While the child is exhaling, activate the MDI by pressing down to release the medication into the spacer device. Tell the child to take 3-5 slow, deep breaths, holding the last one for 10 seconds.
    - **Lung tissue disease** pg. 134 **-** pneumonia, pulmonary edema, or ARDS. S/S: **grunting**, crackles, hypercarbia. TX: high-flow nasal cannula, CPAP, mechanical ventilation with PEEP.
    - **Disordered control of breathing** pg. 137 – seizures, head injury, increased ICP, hydrocephalus, neuromuscular disorders, drug overdose.

        - **Increased ICP** pg. 137 – irregular breathing is a component of Cushing's triad. TX: ensure head is midline, administer osmotic diuretics or hypertonic saline, treat agitation and pain, avoid hypotension.
    - **Management of Respiratory/Failure Flowchart pg. 141**
    - **Bag-Mask Ventilation** pgs. 142-152
        - E-C clamp one and two-person technique, ventilate at a rate of **1 breath every 2-3 seconds**, deliver each breath over 1 second, and monitor for **visible chest rise**.
    - **Positioning of child** to open airway pgs. 147-148 – towel under the shoulders in infants and young child, towel under the occiput for children > age 2 to achieve **"sniffing" position**.
    - **Oropharyngeal airway (OPA)** insertion pg. 154 – measure from corner of the mouth to the angle of the jaw. Use a tongue blade to depress the tongue and insert the OPA.
    - **Sudden deterioration in an Intubated Patient (DOPE Mnemonic) pg.** 163 - **D** – Displacement, **O** – Obstruction, **P** – Pneumothorax, **E** – Equipment failure.
- **Shock – Chapters 9 & 10**
    - **Shock** can result from low blood volume (hypovolemic), maldistribution of blood flow (distributive), impaired contractility (cardiogenic), or obstructed blood flow.
    - **Compensated shock** pg. 171 – signs of poor perfusion, but a **normal systolic blood pressure**.
        - S/S: tachycardia, cool, pale, diaphoretic skin, **weak peripheral pulses**, **narrow pulse pressure** (not hypotension), oliguria, restlessness, vomiting.
    - **Hypotensive shock** – weak or absent distal pulses, altered LOC, **hypotension**.
    - **Hypovolemic shock** pg. 174 – vomiting, diarrhea, hemorrhage, fluid loss.
    - **Distributive shock** pg. 175 – maldistribution of blood flow, relative hypovolemia.
        - **Septic shock** pg. 177 – **flash capillary refill in early sepsis**, petechial or purpuric rash, anxiety.
        - **Anaphylactic shock** pg. 179 – angioedema, **respiratory distress with stridor**, urticarial (hives) rash, nausea, and vomiting.
        - **Neurogenic shock** pg. 180 – loss of sympathetic tone, lack of tachycardia and peripheral vasoconstriction, hypothermia.
    - **Cardiogenic shock** pg. 180 – pump failure from congenital heart disease, myocarditis, cardiomyopathy, myocardial injury.
    - **Obstructive shock** pgs. 183-185 – pericardial tamponade, tension pneumothorax, ductal-dependent heart defects, massive pulmonary embolism.
        - **Cardiac tamponade** pg. 183 – diminished heart sounds, pulsus paradoxus.
        - **Tension pneumothorax** pg. 184 – respiratory distress, diminished or absent breath sounds, tracheal deviation, pulsus paradoxus.
        - **Left ventricular outflow lesions** pg. 186 – congestive heart failure, absent or weaker femoral pulses (coarctation).
    - **Recognizing Shock Flowchart pg. 188**
    - The **goal of shock treatment** is to improve perfusion, optimize oxygen delivery to the cells, reduce oxygen demand, and correct metabolic derangements. Treat **hypoglycemia** and metabolic acidosis.
    - **Laboratory Studies** pg. 195 – **Lactate** is a product of anaerobic metabolism.
    - Vasoactive Therapy used in Treating Shock pg. 197 – Inotropes, inodilators (Milrinone), vasodilators, vasopressors (Epinephrine, Norepinephrine, Vasopressin)
    - **Fluid resuscitation in Shock** pgs. 198-201 – **isotonic crystalloid bolus of 20 mL/kg** over 5 to 20 minutes (**5 to 10 minutes for hypovolemic shock**), reassess after each bolus, and repeat as needed. **Administer 10-20 mL/kg is sepsis**, may require 60 mL/kg during the first hour.
    - Fluid guide on pg. 201. **Transfuse blood products at 10 mL/kg for hemorrhage.**
    - **Managing glucose** pg. 204 – **2-4 mL/kg of D 25%** or 5-10 mL/kg of D 10%.
    - Nonhemorrhagic hypovolemic shock pgs. 206-207 – stages of dehydration.
    - Hemorrhagic hypovolemic shock pgs. 207-209 – blood loss chart. Control hemorrhage, infuse, and transfuse.
    - **Pediatric Septic Shock Algorithm pg. 211** – draw labs and blood culture, **administer antibiotics.**
    - **Anaphylactic Shock pg. 216** – Place patient in a supine position, administer oxygen, maintain airway. IM epinephrine, isotonic fluids, albuterol, antihistamines, corticosteroids.

- **Management of Shock Flowchart pg. 222**
- **Intraosseous Access** pgs. 223-226
  - Reduce pain of intraosseous infusion with plain xylocaine.

- **Pediatric Cardiac Arrhythmias - Chapters 11 & 12,** Cardiac Rhythms pgs. 290-293
  - **Bradycardia Algorithm pg. 244** – CPR if HR < 60/minute despite oxygenation and ventilation. Epinephrine and possibly Atropine.
  - **Tachycardia Algorithm pg. 257.** Tachycardias pgs. 236-240. **Vagal maneuver** pg. 250 – ice to upper half of face for 15 to 20 seconds. **Medications to treat tachycardias** pgs. 251-52 – Adenosine and Amiodarone.
  - **Synchronized Cardioversion** pg. 253-256 – for hemodynamically **unstable tachycardic** patients (poor perfusion, hypotension, heart failure) with a pulse. Start with an energy dose of **0.5 to 1 J/kg, increase to 2 J/kg**.
- **Post-Cardiac Arrest Care – Chapter 13**
  - Checklist pg. 263 – **oxygen saturation 94-99%**, $ETCO_2$ 35-45 mm Hg
  - **Management of Shock after ROSC Algorithm pg. 271**
  - Maintenance fluid calculation pg. 274 (4-2-1 Method)

Pediatric Primary Survey (ABCDE) with (FG)

- Airway and Alertness (AVPU)
  - Neck in **neutral position, padding under shoulders**
- Breathing and Ventilation
  - Confirm tube size with resuscitation tape
  - Decompress the stomach with a gastric tube
- Circulation and Control of Hemorrhage
  - Normal capillary refill is 2 seconds or less
  - **20 ml/kg fluid bolus over 5-10 minutes**
    - **Pull-push with 3-way stopcock**
    - 5-10 ml/kg over 10-20 minutes for cardiogenic shock
  - Blood/blood products at 10 ml/kg after 2 boluses if blood loss
- Disability "Da Brain"
  - Pediatric Glasgow Coma Scale – airway for GCS 8 or less
  - PERRL and **check glucose**
- Exposure and Environmental Control
- Full set of vitals and Family Presence
  - Hypotension = < 60 SBP in neonate, < 70 in infant, 70 + (2 x age in years) for 1-10 age
  - Widened pulse pressure in early septic shock or increased ICP; Narrow PP in early hypotensive shock
  - **Weight in kg's only**
  - Assess the needs of the family
- Get adjuncts and Give comfort
  - L = Labs (bedside glucose)
  - M = Monitor
  - N = Nasogastric (**contraindicated in head and facial injury**) or OG consideration
  - O = Oxygenation (PO) and **ET CO_2 capnography**
  - P = Pain assessment and management

Triage Process (20 Exam Questions) (Refer to Chapter 4 in 6th edition ENPC or Chapter 11 in 5th edition ENPC)

- The **Pediatric Assessment Triangle** (PAT) – Across-the-room Assessment
  - **Appearance**
    - **TICLS - T**one, **I**nteractiveness, **C**onsolability, **L**ook/gaze, **S**peech/cry.
  - **Work of Breathing** – tachypnea or bradypnea, tripoding, retractions, nasal flaring, head-bobbing, abnormal breath sounds.
  - **Circulation to the Skin** – pale, mottled, ashen, gray, dusky, or cyanotic skin.
- **Sick, Sicker, Sickest**
  - Sick (no disruption of PAT), Sicker (one disruption of PAT), Sickest (two or more disruptions of PAT).
- **ESI Triage** 5-level triage based on initial presentation – download free ESI 5th edition on ENA University app.
  - Level 1 requires immediate life-saving intervention, level 2 is high-risk (ex: sickle cell crisis, testicular torsion, suicidal, ectopic pregnancy), levels 3 to 5 based on anticipated resources (level 5 requires no resources, level 4 requires one resource, level 3 requires 2 or more resources).
- Isolation Concerns – obtain a vaccine and exposure history. Skin rash with abnormal PAT may require isolation.
- Risk for Harm – ask child if they have suicidal thoughts, use a **suicide screening tool**, triage as level 2.
  - "Have you ever wished you were dead?"
  - "Have you ever felt your family would be better off if you were dead?"
  - "Do you have thoughts of killing yourself?" "If so, do you think about how you might do this?"
  - "Have you ever acted on these thoughts?"
- **Sexual Orientation and Gender Identity**
  - Gender identity may be different than sex assigned at birth.
  - Sexual attraction may be heterosexual, homosexual, bisexual, pansexual, or asexual.
  - Inquire, "How may I best address you?"
- **Disaster Decontamination** in Pediatrics
  - Children are more vulnerable to toxins since higher respiratory rate and inhale more airborne gases, they have thinner skin so absorb more toxins. Children may also hide from rescuers.
  - Keep families together or reunite quickly, keep child war, during decontamination.
  - Hot zone for those in appropriate attire, life-saving care only. Warm zone for decontamination with soap and water. Cold zone for treatment.
- **Mass Casualty Disaster Triage** (Chapter 4 in 6th edition ENPC. Chapter 31 in 5th edition ENPC)
  - **START Triage** is based on RPM – **R**espiration (< 15 or >45 in pediatrics), **P**erfusion (capillary refill > 2 seconds), and **M**ental status (P or U on AVPU).
  - **JumpSTART** is for infants and children up to 8 years of age. Provide 5 positive-pressure breaths before moving to black tarp if the patient has a pulse.
  - **Red** tag is emergent/immediate, **Yellow** tag is urgent/delayed, **Green** tag is walking wounded/nonurgent, **Black** tag is deceased/expectant to die.

Assessment (25 Exam Questions) (Refer to Chapter 5 in 6th edition ENPC or Chapter 6 in 5th edition ENPC)

- Preparation – length-based resuscitation tape, assign roles, pediatric-sized equipment, consider safety threats and need for decontamination.
- **Initial Assessment** –A-J Mnemonic for standardized systematic approach
- **Primary Survey**
  - **A**lertness and **A**irway
    - AVPU – **A**lert, responsive to **V**erbal stimuli, responsive to **P**ainful stimuli, **U**nresponsive
    - Sniffing position – padding under shoulders and upper torso.
    - Head-tilt or jaw-thrust maneuver.
    - Oral airway (OPA) – measure from the corner of the mouth to the angle of the jaw, use a tongue blade and slide OPA directly over tongue, do not turn the OPA.
  - **B**reathing and Ventilation
    - Assess breathing effectiveness and listen to midaxillary breath sounds.
    - Assist breathing with a bag-mask device if needed.
    - If intubated, auscultate over epigastrium and bilateral lungs, use continuous waveform capnography.
    - Secure the tube and note the measurement at the gums or the lips.
  - **C**irculation and **C**ontrol of Hemorrhage
    - Assess capillary refill by blanching the forehead, sole of foot, or palm of hand. Normal capillary refill is less than 2 seconds.
    - 20 mL/kg isotonic crystalloid for hypovolemic shock over 5 to 10 minutes.
    - 10 mL/kg of blood/blood products for hemorrhage.
      - Push-Pull Technique Box 5-2
    - "Stop the Bleed" through direct pressure initially, wound packing, and tourniquets.
  - **D**isability
    - Glasgow Coma Scale Table 5-1
    - PERRL
    - Check blood glucose.
  - **E**xposure and **E**nvironmental Control
    - Warm blankets, fluids, lights.
  - **F**ull set of vital signs and **F**amily presence
    - Hypotension = < 60 SBP in neonate, < 70 in infant, 70 + (2 x age in years) for 1-10 age.
    - Narrow pulse pressure seen in early hypotensive shock.
    - Weight in kilograms only.
  - **G**et adjuncts and **G**ive comfort.
    - **L**aboratory analysis (blood glucose)
    - **M**onitor (cardiac, NIBP)
    - **N**asogastric or orogastric tube to reduce the risk of aspiration and improve tidal volume.
    - **O**xygenation and capnography
    - **P**ain assessment and management
- **Secondary Survey**
  - **H**istory (SAMPLE) and **H**ead-to-toe examination
    - SAMPLE – **S**igns and **S**ymptoms, **A**llergies, **M**edications, **P**ast medical history, **L**ast meal, **E**vents leading to current illness or injury.
  - **I**nspect posterior surfaces.
  - **J**ust keep reevaluating.
    - **VIPP** – **V**ital signs, **I**dentified abnormalities, **P**rimary survey, **P**ain.

- **Children with Special Needs** (Chapter 18 in 6th edition ENPC)
  - **Cerebral Palsy** – a neuromuscular disorder characterized by movement limitations and spasticity, which commonly results from prenatal or postnatal brain injuries. At least 50% of patients are of at least normal intelligence, so include them in your plans of care. Epilepsy is seen in 25to 45% of patients. Intrathecal baclofen pumps are used to decrease spasticity. Baclofen withdrawal may lead to hyperthermia and seizures.
  - **Cystic Fibrosis** – an autosomal recessive condition in which a defective gene alters the ability to regulate sodium and chloride in the body, leading to thick mucoid. Mucus obstruction leads to pneumonia and constipation.
  - **Down Syndrome (Trisomy 21) –** a genetic condition due to an extra chromosome, seen more in pregnancies of women older than 35 years of age. Increased incidence of atlantoaxial instability, take care in cervical spinal precautions.
  - **Marfan Syndrome** – a connective tissue disorder causing aortic dilation and aneurysms, spontaneous pneumothorax, and atlantoaxial subluxation.
  - **Osteogenesis Imperfecta "Brittle Bone"** – do not lift the patient's ankles to change a diaper, lift using one hand under the buttocks and one hand under the head.
- **Pain**
  - Revised FLACC scale 0 to 10 (Table 3-5) is useful for nonverbal patients, assesses face, legs, activity, cry, and consolability.
  - Wong-Baker FACES scale for approximately **age 8**.
  - Nonpharmacologic interventions – distraction (blowing bubbles, videos, singing), non-nutritive sucking, caregiver presence, and warmth. Ice may cause hypothermia.
  - Pharmacologic Interventions (Table 3-6)
    - **Ketamine**
      - Can be administered intranasal, intramuscular, or intravenous.
      - Rapid onset and half-life 2.5 hours.
      - Provides sedation, analgesia, and amnesia without respiratory depression.
      - Contraindicated in under 3 months of age.
      - Emergence reaction is rare.

System-Focused Emergencies (56 Exam Questions)

- **Respiratory Emergencies** (Refer to Chapter 8 in 5th or 6th edition ENPC)
    - **Respiratory distress** – tachypnea, nasal flaring, retractions, pallor, irritability, tripod.
    - Progresses to **Respiratory failure** – bradypnea to apnea, bradycardia, altered LOC (**lethargy),** head bobbing, hypoxia despite oxygenation.
    - **Bag-Mask Ventilation** PALS pgs. 142-152
        - E-C clamp one and two-person technique, ventilate 5-7 mL/kg tidal volume at a rate of **1 breath every 2-3 seconds**, deliver each breath over 1 second, and monitor for **visible chest rise**.
    - **Positioning of child** to open airway PALS pgs. 147-148 – towel under the shoulders in infants and young child, towel under the occiput for children > age 2 to achieve **"sniffing" position**.
    - Tracheal intubation with a **cuffed ET tube** is recommended, colorimetric device should turn **yellow**.
    - **Oropharyngeal airway (OPA)** insertion PALS pg. 154 – measure from corner of the mouth to the angle of the jaw. Use a tongue blade to depress the tongue and insert the OPA.
    - **Sudden deterioration in an Intubated Patient (DOPE Mnemonic)** PALS pg. 163 - **D** – Displacement, **O** – Obstruction, **P** – Pneumothorax, **E** – Equipment failure.
    - **Tracheostomy** – pediatric tracheostomy tubes are shorter and typically do not have an inner cannula.
    - **Foreign body** – more common in children < age 2, complaint of choking causing sudden onset of respiratory distress, may require bronchoscopy.
    - Congenital conditions
        - Tracheomalacia is a tracheal cartilage collapse (pg. 95).
        - Cystic fibrosis (6th edition pg. 281) – thick mucus leads to pneumonia.
    - Upper airway obstruction
        - **Croup (laryngotracheitis)** is caused by a respiratory virus.
            - S/S: Stridor, barking cough that worsens at night, low-grade fever, steeple sign on x-ray.
            - TX: Corticosteroids and nebulized epinephrine for moderate to severe croup.
            - D/C instructions: Cool mist humidifier or steamy bathroom.
        - **Epiglottitis** is commonly caused by *Hemophilus influenzae* type B.
            - S/S: 3 D's – **D**ysphagia, **d**rooling, and respiratory **d**istress, stridor, "hot potato" muffled voice, tripod positioning, high fever.
            - TX: Airway management and oxygen (consult an airway specialist). Labs and antibiotics are held until the airway is secure since crying may occlude airway.
        - **Inhalation** injuries – children are more sensitive to the effects of **carbon monoxide** (CO) poisoning due to increased respiratory rates. Treat with high flow oxygen.
        - **Tracheobronchial injury -** blunt injury from "clothesline-type" injury, positive-pressure ventilation may increase subcutaneous emphysema.
    - Lower airway obstruction
        - **Bronchiolitis** – commonly caused by respiratory syncytial virus (RSV) in children < age 2 with exposure to smoking or daycare attendance.
            - S/S: cough that worsens with crying, tachypnea, retractions, wheezing and crackles, pallor, low oxygen saturation.
            - TX: nasal suctioning and high-flow nasal cannula.
        - **Pneumonia**
            - S/S: fever, cough, tachypnea, increased work of breathing.
            - TX: early antibiotics.

- **Asthma**
    - S/S: cough, wheezing, tachypnea, prolonged expiratory phase, accessory muscle use, retractions; a silent chest is a red flag.
    - DX: measure peak expiratory flow rate (green, yellow, red) before and after medical management to gauge improvement.
    - TX: oxygen, inhaled short-acting beta agonists including albuterol (salbutamol) and levalbuterol, oral or intravenous corticosteroids, nebulized ipratropium (anticholinergic), nebulized or intravenous magnesium, Heliox, ketamine for sedation prior to intubation since it is a bronchodilator.
    - D/C instructions: Instructions on peak flow meter to establish "personal best" and inhaler with spacer.

- **Cardiovascular Emergencies** (Refer to Chapter 9 in 5th or Chapter 7 in 6th edition ENPC)
  - **Pericarditis** – inflammation of the pericardial sac.
    - S/S: pleuritic retrosternal chest pain, **worse with inspiration and supine position**.
    - DX: global concave ST segment elevation on EKG. A friction rub is best heard at the left sternal border with diaphragm.
    - TX: NSAIDS and allow to lean forward. Monitor for cardiac tamponade.
  - **Congenital heart defects (CHD)** – (see neonatal emergencies)
  - **Rhythm disturbances** (Table 7-4 in 6th edition ENPC)
    - **Bradycardia with a pulse**
      - Treat reversible causes such as hypoxia with positive-pressure ventilation.
      - Atropine is only used if bradycardia is the result of an AV block.
      - CPR if HR < 60/minute despite oxygenation and ventilation.
      - Epinephrine.
      - Consider pacing.
    - **Sinus Tachycardia** – treat the cause.
    - **Tachycardia with a pulse** (Consult cardiology)
      - **Stable Supraventricular Tachycardia (SVT)** (> 220 in infant, > 180 in child)
        - Vagal maneuver – ice to upper half of face for 15 to 20 seconds.
        - Adenosine SLAM.
      - **Unstable SVT -** Synchronized Cardioversion at an energy dose of 0.5 to 1 J/kg, increase to 2 J/kg.
    - **Stable Ventricular Tachycardia (VT)** (rate 120 to 200 beats/minute, wide QRS)
      - Adenosine if rhythm is regular monomorphic QRS.
      - Amiodarone over 20 to 60 minutes.
      - **Unstable VT -** Synchronized Cardioversion at an energy dose of 0.5 to 1 J/kg, increase to 2 J/kg. May give an unsynchronized shock to unstable patients.
  - **Cardiac arrest** (PALS pgs. 89-92)
    - CPR at a rate of 100 to 120 compressions per minute.
    - Epinephrine every 4 minutes.
    - Shockable rhythm - Defibrillate at 2-4 J/kg, up to 10 J/kg. Use infant pads for < 10 kg or younger than 1 year. "Clear for shock". Administer amiodarone or lidocaine.
    - Consider the cause of arrest – Hs and Ts.
    - Post-Resuscitation
      - Optimize airway, breathing, and circulation, while avoiding hyperoxia and hyperthermia. Administer maintenance intravenous fluids.

- **Shock** (Refer to Chapter 10 in 5th or Chapter 7 in 6th edition ENPC)
    - Shock physiology - sympathetic nervous system is stimulated causing the release of catecholamines epinephrine and norepinephrine yielding vasoconstriction and increased contractility.
    - **Stages of Shock** (Table 7-1)
        - Compensated – tachycardia, mild tachypnea, slightly delayed capillary refill, subtle change in mental status, narrowed pulse pressure.
        - Hypotensive (decompensated) – altered mental status, pallor, hypotension.
        - Irreversible – bradycardia, unresponsive.
    - **Shock types** (Table 7-5)
        - **Hypovolemic** – the most common form of shock.
            - **Hemorrhagic** hypovolemic shock
                - "Stop the bleed" – direct pressure, packing, tourniquets.
                - Blood/blood product replacement at 10 mL/kg
            - **Non-hemorrhagic** hypovolemic shock
                - Isotonic crystalloid bolus of 20 mL/kg over 5 to 10 minutes reassess after each bolus and repeat as needed. Patient may require 60 mL/kg during the first hour.
        - **Cardiogenic** – pump failure, decreased cardiac contractility and output.
            - Isotonic crystalloid bolus of 5-10 ml/kg slowly over 10-30 minutes.
            - Vasopressors or inotropic medications.
        - **Obstructive** – physical obstruction of blood flow.
            - **Cardiac tamponade** – fluid in pericardial sac.
                - Beck's triad – hypotension, muffled heart sounds, and jugular vein distention.
            - **Tension pneumothorax** – air in pleural cavity collapses alveoli, from trauma, spontaneous, or vaping.
                - Tachycardia, respiratory distress, hypotension, jugular vein distention, tracheal deviation.
            - **Pulmonary embolism** – blockage of the pulmonary arteries, from a blood clot, fat emboli, or air embolus. Risk factors include obesity, hormone use, hypercoagulopathy, prolonged immobility, surgery, or trauma. Treatment includes anticoagulation., fibrinolysis, or thrombectomy.
        - **Distributive** – maldistribution with systemic vasodilation, yielding a relative hypovolemia.
            - **Neurogenic** - unopposed parasympathetic nervous system stimulation leads to bradycardia and vasodilation.
                - S/S: spinal cord injury; bradycardia, bradypnea, hypotension.
                - TX: IV fluid and increase vascular tone with vasopressors and inotropes.
            - **Septic** – endotoxin release
                - Early S/S – bounding pulses, flash capillary refill (< 1 second).
                - TX: Isotonic crystalloid bolus of 10 to 20 mL/kg up to 40 to 60 mL/kg over the first hour. Infuse epinephrine or norepinephrine, and antibiotics within 1 hour of ED arrival.
            - **Anaphylactic** – an overwhelming allergic reaction.
                - S/S: hives, flushing, airway swelling, respiratory distress, stridor, urticaria, wheezing, vomiting, and diarrhea.
                - TX: priority is Epinephrine IM in lateral thigh (vastus lateralis), inhaled albuterol, histamine blockers (diphenhydramine, famotidine), steroids.

- **Circulatory support**
  - Vascular access – Secure with a **transparent** dressing so see subtle signs of infiltration, never wrap an IV or IO line circumferentially. (ENPC 6th pg. 37)
  - Extracorporeal membrane oxygenation (ECMO) may be used for the critically ill child not responding to epinephrine or norepinephrine. (ENPC 6th pg. 155)
  - Ventricular assist device (VAD) – faint peripheral pulses are expected, obtain blood pressure with doppler.
- **Chest Trauma** (ENPC 6th pg. 142)
  - **Pneumothorax** – a collection of air in the pleural space (air leak syndrome). S/S: decreased or absent breath sounds on the affected side and hyperresonance on percussion..
  - **Hemothorax** – a collection of blood in the pleural space. S/S: tachycardia, pale and cool skin, respiratory distress, dullness on percussion. TX: chest tube and treat shock.
  - **Tension pneumothorax** – air cannot escape on expiration, intrathoracic pressure increases, causing obstructive shock. S/S: dyspnea, absent or reduced breath sounds on injured side, tracheal shift away from injured side. TX: needle decompression/thoracostomy and chest tube insertion.
  - **Rib fractures** – high risk for underlying thoracic and abdominal solid-organ injuries due to cartilaginous thoracic cage. Consider child maltreatment with rib fractures.

- **Neurological Emergencies** (Refer to Chapter 15 in 5th or Chapter 14 in 6th edition ENPC)
  - **Meningitis** – Prevent bacterial infection with HIB immunization.
    - S/S in infants: irritability, inconsolability, shrill cry, and tense or bulging fontanelle.
    - S/S in children: fever, headache, nuchal rigidity, phonophobia, and photophobia.
    - DX: lumbar puncture in side-lying position (oxygen during procedure, monitor respiratory status).
    - TX: Isolation is priority, fluid boluses, and antibiotics.
  - **Hydrocephalus** – overproduction of or obstruction of cerebral spinal fluid (CSF)
    - S/S infants: irritability, higher-pitched cry, widening cranial sutures, bulging fontanelles, vomiting, sleepiness, "sun-setting" eyes.
    - S/S children: vomiting, headache, vision changes, gait abnormalities.
    - DX: monitor head circumference, brain MRI.
    - TX: elevate HOB, drain shunt, antibiotics.
  - **Ventriculoperitoneal VP/ Ventriculoatrial VA Shunt dysfunction** - VP shunt diverts the CSF from the ventricles to the peritoneum, VA to right atrium of heart.
  - **Headache** – Red flags are "thunderclap", ataxia, fever.
    - Tension – bilateral dull pain.
    - Migraine – sharp, pulsating pain associated with nausea and vomiting, phonophobia and photophobia.
    - TX: ibuprofen, antiemetics.
  - **Seizures** (ENPC 6th Figure 14-4)
    - Causes: toxins, hypoglycemia, electrolyte imbalance, formula dilution, fever.
    - S/S: bicycling of legs and lip-smacking in infants.
    - Status epilepticus – continuous tonic-clonic seizure for 5 minutes or greater.
      - TX: Place patient on side to prevent aspiration and protect head, administer Midazolam IM or IN if no IV access, Lorazepam or Midazolam IV/IO first-line management. 2nd line includes Levetiracetam (Keppra), valproic acid, phenytoin (Dilantin) over 20 minutes, or fosphenytoin (Cerebryx).

- **Stroke** –increased risk of ischemic stroke in patients with sickle cell disease, increased risk of hemorrhagic stroke in patients with AV malformation.
    - S/S of ischemic stroke: speech and visual disturbances, dysphagia (difficulty swallowing), ataxia.
  - S/S of hemorrhagic stroke: sudden onset of headache and vomiting, with rapid deterioration.
  - Consult neurology and obtain a brain MRI.
- **Head Trauma** (ENPC 6th edition pgs. 136-140)
  - S/S: of increased intracranial pressure (ICP) – altered mental status, bulging or tense fontanelle, ecchymosis with basilar skull fractures, CSF leakage (halo test). Missed in infancy due to open fontanelles.
  - TX: of increased ICP – elevate head of bed and keep head midline to facilitate drainage, avoid hyperthermia, hypoxia, and hypotension, administer Mannitol or hypertonic saline, sedation, and anticonvulsants.
  - **Concussion** (mild traumatic brain injury) Follow **CDC "HEADS Up" Program** (Figure 9-6)
    - DC instructions: acetaminophen only, no NSAIDs or narcotics for pain, physical and cognitive rest, 6-step graduated return-to-play protocol (Box 9-2) until baseline balance and cognitive performance.
    - Secondary impact syndrome – repeated head injuries may cause death.
  - **Epidural Hematoma** – injury to temporal area tearing the middle meningeal arterial so rapid bleed. S/S: Headache, vomiting without nausea, possible lucid period.
  - **Subdural Hematoma** – venous bleed so steady decline in LOC, irritability, seizures. Consider maltreatment from shaken impact (abusive brain injury).

- **Gastrointestinal Emergencies** (Refer to Chapter 18 in 5th or Chapters 11 and 12 in 6th edition ENPC)
  - **Foreign body** – keep patient NPO, consult a pediatric gastroenterologist, prepare for endoscopy.
    - Button batteries emit electrical discharge and cause tissue erosion.
    - Magnets cause pressure necrosis, bowel obstruction, and perforation.
    - Body packing – illicit drug smuggling, packets may rupture.
    - Superabsorbent polymers – expand in the stomach, may lead to bowel obstruction or perforation.
    - Fishing weights can lead to acute lead poisoning.
  - **Appendicitis**
    - S/S: fever, nausea, vomiting, anorexia, periumbilical to RLQ abdominal pain at McBurney's point, with rebound tenderness and guarding, psoas sign (flex thigh at hip).
    - TX: NPO, IV antibiotics, monitor WBC (shift to the left), probable surgery.
  - **Pyloric Stenosis**
    - S/S: projectile, non-bilious vomiting after feeding, with continual hunger and weight loss, palpable olive-shaped mass with visible peristaltic waves. May require pyloromyotomy.
  - **Intussusception** (telescoping bowel)
    - Increased risk with celiac and Crohn's, 3-26 months.
    - S/S: intermittent severe colicky pain and inconsolability, drawing up legs to chest, sausage-shaped mass, and currant jelly-like stool.
    - TX: air or contrast enema with ultrasound guidance.
  - **Volvulus** (malrotation)
    - S/S: bilious vomiting with abdominal distention. Surgical emergency.
  - **Inflammatory Bowel Disease (IBD)**
    - Crohn's affects the entire GI system and ulcerative colitis affects the colon only. Meckel's diverticulum – painless GI bleeding with maroon-colored stools.
    - S/S: Bloody diarrhea or frequent loose stools.

- **Abdominal Trauma**
    - **Liver** – right upper quadrant (RUQ) pain with ecchymosis of the umbilical area. Prepare for MTP and damage control surgery.
    - **Spleen** – left upper quadrant (LUQ) pain radiating to the left shoulder (Kehr's sign).
    - **Hollow organs/Bowel rupture** – lap belt injury.

- **Genitourinary and Obstetric Emergencies** (Refer to Chapter 19 in 5th edition ENPC)
  - **Chlamydia** – mucopurulent discharge, common cause of epididymitis. Treat with doxycycline or azithromycin.
  - **Gonorrhea** – mucopurulent discharge, dyspareunia. Treat with ceftriaxone.
  - **Syphilis** – serology testing. Treat with penicillin. Long term neurological and cardiovascular effects.
  - **Herpes** – painful genital lesions. Treat with antivirals.
  - **Epididymitis** – gradual onset of scrotal pain, erythema, and dysuria. Scrotal elevation may decrease pain.
  - **Testicular torsion** – sudden onset of severe unilateral scrotal pain and swelling with absent cremasteric reflex. Immediate urologic consult for detorsion or surgery.
  - **Priapism** - painful penile erection. Evaluate blood flow and urgent urology consultation.
  - **Ovarian torsion -** sudden onset of RLQ pain (appendicitis mimic) in adolescent females, surgical emergency.
  - **Ectopic pregnancy** – pain referred to shoulder and vaginal bleeding 6 to 8 weeks post last menstrual period. TX: Methotrexate or surgery, blooding typing for Rh. Pregnancy loss support.
  - **Urethral (straddle) injury** – blood at the urinary meatus, hematuria. Place a suprapubic catheter.
- **Maxillofacial, Ocular, ENT Emergencies** (Refer to Chapter 17 in 5th edition ENPC)
  - **Maxillary** facial fractures (Le Fort) I – lip laceration, maxillary fracture; II – nasal fracture, pyramid fracture; III – complete craniofacial dissociation. Facial fracture D/C instructions: avoid straining, bending over, heavy lifting, and blowing nose. **Mandibular fracture** – malocclusion, paresthesia of lower lip and jaw.
  - **Avulsed permanent tooth** – rinse gently for 10 seconds without touching root (hold by crown), store in calcium-based solution such as milk.
  - **Orbital fracture** – periorbital edema, hyperesthesia of the cheek and upper lip, limited upward gaze.
  - **Ocular burn** – alkaline (cement, lye, lime, ammonia) injuries are more severe, irrigate with warm NS or LR until normal pH of 7.0 to 7.4. No eye patching.
  - **Eyelid laceration –** ESI triage level 3 due to consulting ophthalmology to assess ocular injury. Consult plastic surgery to repair if full thickness laceration.
  - **Penetrating ocular injury** – use paper cup to stabilize foreign body.
  - **Hyphema –** blood in anterior chamber, keep head of bed at least 30 degrees, cover eye with rigid shield to protect. Increased risk of rebleed in 3-5 days.
  - **Globe rupture** – eye pain, impaired vision, tear-drop shaped pupil. Place a rigid protective eye shield, requires surgical repair.
  - **Conjunctivitis** – Eyelids crusted shut. Apply warm compresses and wash hands after touching eyes.
  - **Epistaxis**– hold head down and pinch nares. Administer phenylephrine (not cocaine) for vasoconstriction.
  - **Nasal foreign bodies** – "Parent's kiss".
  - **Ear foreign bodies** - use lukewarm water for ear irrigation, suction, or Katz extractor. Viscous xylocaine or mineral oil to kill insects, then suction out. Flashlight in dark room to attract flying insects. (Least invasive).
  - **Pharyngitis –** obtain rapid strep screen.
  - **Peritonsillar abscess** – fever, sore throat, "hot potato voice". Prepare for aspiration.
  - **Otitis externa** – pain upon palpation of tragus, keep ear canal dry.
  - **Otitis media** – complete antibiotics.

- **Musculoskeletal Emergencies** (Refer to Chapter 20 in 5th edition ENPC)
  - **Osteogenesis Imperfecta** (brittle bones) – do not lift by ankles to change diaper.
  - **Legg-Calve-Perthes disease** – avascular necrosis of the femoral head, most in shorter stature of 4-8-year-old boys. May present with a limp and decreased range of motion.
  - **Slipped Capital Femoral Epiphysis** – hip disorder seen in early adolescence, especially if **obese**. TX: non-weight bearing, ortho referral.
  - **Juvenile Idiopathic Arthritis** – morning stiffness, arthralgia, fever. TX: NSAIDs and therapy.
  - **Duchenne Muscular Dystrophy** – gait disturbances, progressive weakness. Support breathing.
  - **Epiphyseal-metaphyseal (Salter-Harris)** fractures involve the growth plate.
  - **Greenstick** fractures do not fully break.
  - **Radial head subluxation** – due to sudden jerk on arm. Refuses use of the affected extremity.
  - **Crush injury** – monitor for compartment syndrome (may require fasciotomy), and rhabdomyolysis (dark, tea-colored urine is myoglobinuria).
  - **Compartment Syndrome** – hallmark sign is pain disproportionate to injury on passive movement, despite analgesia. Pulselessness is a late sign. Keep extremity in neutral position (at level of the heart), prepare for a fasciotomy.
  - **Amputation** – apply a tourniquet of stump for bleed control. Gently rinse the amputated part, wrap in saline-moistened gauze. Keep the amputated part on top of ice, do not let it freeze.
- **Integumentary Emergencies** (Refer to Chapter 13 in 6th edition ENPC)
  - **Henoch-Schoenlein Purpura (HSP)** – IgA vasculitis from overactive immune response to respiratory illness. The four hallmark complaints are arthritis, GI complaints, kidney inflammation, and a non-blanchable macular-petechial rash on lower extremities and buttocks. Monitor renal function closely.
  - **Immune Thrombocytopenia Purpura (ITP)** – Autoimmune response causing petechiae on the lower extremities and unexplained bruising preceded by a viral illness. Treatment includes IVIG and corticosteroids.
  - **Kawasaki Disease** – Vasculitis affecting the coronary arteries, leading to aneurysms, heart failure, and cardiac dysrhythmias. Morbilliform (resembles measles) rash on torso, fever for at least 5 days, "strawberry tongue", desquamation of skin on fingers and toes, conjunctivitis. Treatment includes IVIG, aspirin, and corticosteroids.
  - **Stevens-Johnson Syndrome (SJS)/Toxic Epidermal Necrolysis (TEN)** – Hypersensitivity medication reaction (allopurinol, sulfa drugs) causing dermal necrosis. Initial S/S include malaise, fever, cough, sore throat, and painful erythematous lesions.
  - **Roseola Infantum** – Blanching papules, fever, sore throat, and conjunctivitis from herpes virus.
  - **Fifth Disease (Erythema Infectiosum)** – "Slapped cheek" rash, fever, runny nose, sore throat caused by parvovirus B19.
  - **Varicella (Chickenpox)** – Vesicular rash appears as "dewdrops on a rose petal" that progress to itchy fluid-filled blisters, then crusted papules. Treat with antihistamines and topical calamine lotion. Place patient on standard, contact, and airborne isolation.
  - **Hand, Foot, and Mouth Disease** – Maculopapular or papulovesicular rash on the hands and soles, with oral ulcers. Educate caregivers on hand hygiene and disinfection of contaminated surfaces.
  - **Impetigo** – Pus-filled vesicles that leave a yellow crust around the nose and mouth.
  - **Scarlet Fever** – Sandpaper-like rash (not on palms and soles) that peels skin after 7 days, Pastia's lines in body creases. Diagnose with strep screen and treat with penicillin. Standard and droplet precautions until 24 hours after the initiation of antibiotics.
  - **Atopic Dermatitis (Eczema)** – Itchy redness and weeping sores. Treatment includes anti-inflammatory agents, bathing with mild soap, and skin hydration.

    - **Scabies** – Pruritic rash on the palms and soles that worsens at night. Treat with permethrin or ivermectin topically, keep on contact isolation. Wash linens and clothing in hot water. Seal un washable items in plastic bag for 72 hours.
    - **Tinea Corporis (Ringworm)** – Well-demarcated, sharply circumscribed oval or circular lesion with a raised edge. Treat with a topical antifungal.
    - **Lice** – Pruritic rash on neck, armpits, waist, and groin. Wash linens and clothing in hot water.
    - **Cimex lectularis (Bed Bugs)** – Bites on arms, legs, face, and neck in clusters of three or more bites. Treat with antihistamine and topical corticosteroids. Wash linens and clothing in hot water.
- **Hematology/Oncology Emergencies** (Refer to Chapter 23 in 5th edition ENPC)
    - **Hemophilia** – Sex-linked congenital coagulation disorder (A–factor VIII, B–factor IX, vWF). TX: Replace clotting factor (cryoprecipitate has factor VII and vWF), blood products if bleeding is severe, aminocaproic acid, DDAVP. If hemarthrosis, elevate, ice, and immobilize affected joints. Avoid aspirin and NSAIDs.
    - **Sickle cell anemia** – Triage sickle cell crisis as ESI level 2, avoid implicit bias. Crisis is triggered by stress, cold, dehydration, or infection. Treat with IVFs to dilute blood and control pain. Hydroxyurea stimulates normal RBC production.
        - Acute chest syndrome – chest pain, dyspnea, cough, hypoxemia; most common cause of death from sickle cell disease. Suspect pulmonary embolus if hemoptysis.
        - Splenic sequestration – LUQ abdominal pain, splenomegaly, hypovolemic shock.
        - Vaso-occlusive crisis – pain in extremities, priapism. Treat with hydration, warm packs over areas of pain.
    - **Neutropenia** (neutrophil < 500) – immune-compromised and unable to fight off infection. Initiate neutropenic precautions – avoid rectal temperatures, exquisite hand hygiene, IV antibiotics. Educate to avoid crowds.
    - **Tumor Lysis Syndrome** – An oncologic emergency seen from the destruction of cells after chemotherapy. Labs: hyperkalemia, hyperuricemia, and hypocalcemia. Treat with fluids and loop diuretics, administer allopurinol to decrease uric acid levels.
- **Endocrine/Metabolic Emergencies** (Refer to Chapter 24 in 5th edition ENPC)
    - **Adrenal insufficiency** from congenital adrenal hyperplasia - hypoglycemia, hyponatremia, and hyperkalemia. Treat with hydrocortisone, dexamethasone, and fluid resuscitation with normal saline.
    - **Hypoglycemia** – blood glucose < 45 mg/dl, 60 for newborn. Administer 10 ml/kg $D_{10}W$ or 2-4 ml/kg $D_{25}W$ if unresponsive.
    - **Diabetic Ketoacidosis (DKA)**
        - S/S: blood glucose > 200 mg/dL or normal blood sugar, pH < 7.3 (anion gap metabolic acidosis), HCO_3 < 15, ketonuria and ketonemia, fruity odor to breath, abdominal pain, signs of profound dehydration, Kussmaul's respirations.
        - TX: IVFs 10-20 ml/kg LR fluid bolus and repeat as needed to treat hypovolemia, replace potassium, insulin infusion (not bolus or cerebral edema) after fluid bolus. Monitor glucose and potassium level closely. Add 5% dextrose when BS 250-300. Infuse Insulin until the anion gap closes (pH > 7.3, HCO_3 > 15).
    - **Diabetes Insipidus (DI)** – ADH deficiency, leads to hyperosmolar dehydration (hypernatremia), shock.
    - **SIADH** – over-secretion of ADH resulting in decreased urine output and dilutional hyponatremia, risk is seizures. Treat with hypertonic saline and treat trigger – head injury or meningitis.

Special Considerations (25 Exam Questions)

- **Neonatal Emergencies** (Refer to Chapter 5 in 5th or Chapter 6 in 6th edition ENPC)
  - **Newborn resuscitation**
    - Warm, dry, and stimulate the neonate.
    - Open the airway and clear the mouth and then the nose with suction bulb syringe.
    - Initiate positive-pressure ventilation (PPV) at 40-60 breaths per minute (most important action).
    - Use **MR SOPA** acronym to ensure ventilation – **M**ask adjustment, **R**eposition head and neck, **S**uction mouth and nose, **O**pen the mouth, **P**ressure increase with PPV, and **A**lternative airway (endotracheal tube).
    - Chest compressions at a rate of 120 compressions per minute with a 3:1 ratio of compressions to ventilations.
    - Fluid resuscitation of 10 mL/kg.
  - **THEMISFITS** mnemonic for abnormal neonatal findings – **T**rauma, **H**eart disease, **E**ndocrine (congenital adrenal hyperplasia), **M**etabolic (hypoglycemia), **I**nborn errors of metabolism, **S**eizures, **F**ormula, **I**ntestinal, **T**oxins, **S**epsis.
  - **NEO SECRETS –** **IN**born errors of metabolism, **E**lectrolyte abnormalities, **O**verdose, **S**eizures, **E**nteric emergencies, **C**ardiac abnormalities, **R**ecipe, **E**ndocrine crisis, **T**rauma, **S**epsis.
  - **TORCH** mnemonic for newborn infections transmitted from the mother – **T**oxoplasmosis, **O**ther (syphilis), **R**ubella (German measles), **C**ytomegalovirus, Herpes.
  - **Congenial Heart Disease (CHD)**
    - S/S: respiratory distress, pulmonary edema, signs of shock, irritability, crying during feedings, decreased activity, poor weight gain.
    - **Cyanotic defects**
      - **Tetralogy of Fallot** – four defects - ventricular septal defect, right ventricular outflow obstruction, and overriding aorta, and right ventricular hypertrophy.
      - **Transposition of great vessels** – severe tachypnea (RR > 60 breaths/minute) without respiratory distress (no retractions or nasal flaring), murmur. Diagnose with echocardiogram. Surgical repair.
    - **Acyanotic defects**
      - **Ventricular septal defect** – the most common defect causing pulmonary edema.
      - **Ductus arteriosum**
        - **Prostaglandin E_1** to prevent closure of ductus - apnea, bradycardia, and hypotension are side effects. Caffeine may be administered to counteract.
      - **Coarctation of the Aorta** – bounding brachial and radial pulses, decreased femoral pulses.
  - **Necrotizing enterocolitis** – vomiting, abdominal distention, and bloody stools. Fluid resuscitation, bowel decompression, antibiotics, and surgical repair.
  - **Congenital diaphragmatic hernia (CDH)** – respiratory distress, scaphoid-shaped abdomen. Insert a gastric tube and prepare for surgical intervention.
  - **Neonatal jaundice** – hyperbilirubinemia causing yellow discoloration of skin (yellow M&M), conjunctiva, and sclera. Increased risk in premature infants and breastfed infants due to early dehydration. Treat with phototherapy.
  - **Neonatal abstinence syndrome** – opioid withdrawal causing irritability, hypertonicity, tremors, vomiting, and diarrhea. Wean opioids gradually.
  - **Phenylketonuria (PKU)** – autosomal recessive gene, unable to process amino acids, musty odor, fair skin, blue eyes, microcephaly. Limit protein, cheese, bread, and aspartame.

- **Behavioral Health Emergencies** (Refer to Chapter 22 in 5th or Chapter 15 in 6th edition ENPC)
  - **Aggressive behavior/De-escalation**
    - Maintain at least two arms lengths away from the agitated patient.
    - Establish rapport, avoid confrontational behavior, maintain a calm facial expression, use active listening.
    - Use clear, simple messages in a soft voice. Explain what will happen in the ED and set limits on unacceptable behavior.
    - Administer oral medications to calm patient, not sedate them.
    - Meet the patient's physical needs.
    - Provide a safe environment, assign a staff member to continuously observe the patient. Remove any harmful objects.
    - Restraints are a last resort to use only when the patient poses an imminent risk to themselves or others.
  - **Depression** – increased due to bullying, gender identity, and technology use, etc.
  - **Suicidal ideation** – ask directly about suicidal ideation (thinking of harming self) or suicide attempt. Risk factors include a family history of suicide, depression, homelessness/runaway, transgender. Utilize a suicidal ideation screening tool.
  - **Post-traumatic stress disorder (PTSD)** – anxiety disorder after a traumatic event. S/S includes nightmares and flashbacks, signs of regression (bedwetting), sleep disturbances, and appetite changes. Maintain consistent staff, ask permission before touching the patient.
  - **Self-injury** – intentional injury (cutting or burning) without suicidal intent. Discuss stress management options.
  - **Eating disorders**
    - **Anorexia nervosa** – a distorted body image, refusal to eat, and disproportionate fear of obesity. S/S includes excessive weight loss, amenorrhea, anemia.
    - **Bulimia nervosa** – compulsion to consume large amounts of food followed by purging through vomiting, use or laxatives or enemas, or excessive exercise. S/S includes calloused hands, erosion of tooth enamel, and gastric erosion.
  - **Agitated delirium** – exacerbation of psychiatric disorders, drug or alcohol intoxication, metabolic imbalance. S/S includes disorientation, hallucinations, incoherent speech, and extreme agitation. Check blood sugar, CBC, ammonia level, and drug screen. Priority is staff and patient safety. Limit stimuli and administer antipsychotic medications.
  - **Bipolar disorder** – euphoria, grandiosity, pressured speech, racing thoughts, and involvement in risky behaviors during mania. Provide a safe environment.
  - **Schizophrenia** – delusions, auditory and visual hallucinations, and disruption in daily functioning emerging in late adolescence to early adulthood. Set limits, do not validate hallucinations. Schizophrenia may be treated with haloperidol, risperidone (Risperdal), olanzapine (Zyprexa).
  - **Antipsychotic extrapyramidal symptoms (EPS)** – dystonia (muscle contraction), akathisia (restlessness), dyskinesia (repetitive movements) – treat with diphenhydramine or benztropine.
  - **Autism spectrum disorders** – place in low stimulus area away from hallways, let caregivers assist, avoid touch as much as possible, maintain consistent team members. Provide noise-cancelling headphones, sunglasses, and a weighted blanket.

- **Maltreatment Emergencies** (Refer to Chapter 13 in 5th or Chapter 16 in 6th edition ENPC)
    - **Forms of Child Maltreatment**
        - Neglect – failure to provide for a child's physical, medical, emotional, or educational needs.
        - Physical abuse – bruises, fractures.
        - Psychological – conveying the child is worthless or unwanted.
        - Sexual abuse – sexual exploitation, trafficking.
        - Medical child maltreatment (Factitious Disorder/Fabricated Illness) – the caregiver's motivation may be a need for attention or to covertly deceive authority figures.
    - **TEN-4-FACES P** – mnemonic for suspicious bruises
        - **T**orso, **E**ar, **N**eck in children under 4 years.
        - **F**renulum, **A**ngle of the jaw/**A**uricular, **C**heeks, **E**yelid, **S**clera in infants under 4 months.
        - **P**atterned injuries.
    - **Abusive head trauma** (Shaken impact) – triad of subdural hemorrhage, retinal hemorrhage, and rib fractures.
    - **Burns** – immersion scald, bilateral/symmetric burn pattern, sharp lines of demarcation, sock or glove-like burn, skinfold sparing genital burns.
    - **Cultural** healing practices – coining, spooning, cupping, moxibustion may be mistaken for abuse.
    - **Conditions mistaken** for child maltreatment – Ehlers-Danlos syndrome (poor weight gain), osteogenesis imperfecta (fractures), Henoch-Schoenlein purpura (symmetrical bruises on the buttocks, arms, legs).
    - **Evaluation** - Ask the child, "what happened?", open-ended questions, document the facts using verbatim words even if vulgar terms are used.
    - **Evidence collection** - avoid cutting off clothes through stains or holes, evidence in separate clean paper bags, follow chain of custody to safeguard evidentiary materials.
- **Environmental Emergencies** (Refer to Chapter 30 in 5th edition ENPC)
    - **Burn Fluid resuscitation formulas.**
        - Fluids prior to BSA calculation
            - 500 ml/hour for 14 and older, 250 ml/hour for 6-13 years of age, 125 ml/hour for 5 years and younger.
        - Based on partial, deep, and full-thickness burns (not superficial).
        - LR is fluid of choice, half of total amount in first 8 hours from time of burn.
        - American Burn Association (ABA) guidelines, ACE it!
            - **A**dult thermal = 2ml x kg x BSA for 24-hour calculation
            - **C**hild thermal = 3ml x kg x BSA for 24-hour calculation (< 14 years of age)
            - **E**lectrical = 4ml x kg x BSA for 24-hour calculation
        - Adjust fluid based on urinary output, need 0.5-1.0 ml/kg/hour adult (30-60 cc/hour), 1-2ml/kg/hour in peds. Infuse D5LR maintenance on pediatric patients to maintain glucose levels.
        - Parkland formula is only **considered** for adult thermal burns= 4ml x kg x BSA for 24-hour calculation.
    - **Electrical burns**
        - Do not document entrance and exit wound, just point of contact. Risk of compartment syndrome due to local tissue injury.
        - Hand-to-hand – increased risk of heart damage since across the heart, risk of V Fib or asystole.
        - Risk of rhabdomyolysis and acute kidney injury so increase IVFs to get UO at least 75-100 ml/hr.
    - **Organophosphate pesticide** toxicity – cholinergic toxidrome. Treatment includes decontamination by washing with soap and water, and atropine and pralidoxime (2-PAM) until bronchial secretions dry.
    - **Carbon Monoxide** – pulse oximetry is unreliable, get carboxyhemoglobin (COHb) levels. Treat with high-flow oxygen.

- **Cyanide** – Treat with hydroxocobalamin (turns urine red since metabolizes into vitamin B12) and sodium thiosulfate.
- **Heat stroke –** cool to 100.4 (38 C) degrees through evaporation, ice packs, fluid resuscitation, and correct electrolyte imbalances.
- **Severe hypothermia** – treat patient with warmed IVFs, heated inspired air, lavage, and/or ECMO.
- **Black widow spider bite** – pinprick followed by muscle abdominal cramps, treat with pain medication and muscle relaxants.
- **Brown recluse spider bite** – painless bite, tissue sloughing, wound care consultation.
- **Lyme disease deer ticks** – erythema migrans, "bullseye" shaped rash, treat with Doxycycline. Facial paralysis possible if untreated.
- **Rocky Mountain Spotted Fever** (Rickettsia) – tick-borne illness 2-5 days after tick bite, nonpruritic maculopapular rash on the wrist and ankles, occasionally on palms and soles.
- **Tick paralysis** – unsteady gait, progressing to ascending symmetrical flaccid paralysis since neurotoxin is like botulinum toxin. Seen more in spring and summer, look for tick. Symptoms similar to Guillain Barre.
- **Rabies –** highest risk from raccoons, foxes, and bats. 60,000 receive post-exposure prophylaxis, only 1-3 cases per year in the US. Administer HRIG 20 units/kg (infiltrate into wound if possible) and vaccine. Symptoms of rabies include hydrophobia, a spasm in throat when swallowing.
- **Pit Viper snakebites** – do not apply ice or tourniquet, administer antivenom if hemorrhagic swelling.
- **Jellyfish sting** – vinegar to inactivate the toxin, flush with hot water.

- **Toxicology** (Refer to Chapter 14 in 6th edition ENPC)
  - **Initial interventions** – donning personal protective equipment (PPE) always takes precedence over patient care. Brush off dry chemicals. Stabilize ABC's.
  - **Acetaminophen** – 150 mg/kg risk of hepatotoxicity, administer charcoal orally within 4 hours of ingestion, N-Acetylcysteine (NAC) within 8 hours of ingestion.
  - **Selective Serotonin Reuptake Inhibitors (SSRIs such as Prozac, Paxil, Zoloft)** – central nervous system depression and seizures. Treat by cooling and with benzodiazepines.
  - **Serotonin syndrome** – hyperthermia, hypertension, tachycardia, and muscle rigidity. Treat with benzodiazepines.
  - **Tricyclic antidepressants (TCAs such as Elavil and Sinequan) -** anticholinergic syndrome – hyperthermia, tachycardia, hypertension, altered mental status, QRS prolongation, ventricular dysrhythmias, seizures. Treat with sodium bicarbonate, lipid emulsion, lidocaine, magnesium, and benzodiazepines.
  - **Benzodiazepines (Xanax and Ativan)** – respiratory and CNS depression. Treatment is supportive, caution using flumazenil (risk is seizures).
  - **Beta and Calcium-channel blockers** – S/S includes bradycardia and hypotension, hypoglycemia in beta-blocker. Treat with IVFs, atropine, calcium, glucagon, vasopressors, pacing, and lipid emulsion.
  - **Iron** (vitamin formulations) – S/S includes vomiting, diarrhea, and gastrointestinal bleeding. An abdominal radiograph may be useful in determining the amount of iron ingested. Treatment includes chelating agent deferoxamine, which turns urine pink as it is excreted.
  - **Opioids** –S/S include respiratory depression with constricted pupils (miosis). Treat with oxygenation and ventilation and consider naloxone. Naloxone is more likely to induce seizures in Tramadol overdose.
  - **Oral hypoglycemics (sulfonylureas, Glucotrol)** – administer dextrose and octreotide.
  - **Salicylates** – S/S includes tinnitus, fever, tachypnea, metabolic acidosis. Treat with fluids and sodium bicarbonate to alkalinize urine.
  - **Ethanol** – monitor for hypoglycemia.
  - **Toxic Alcohols** – methanol, ethylene glycol (antifreeze), and isopropyl alcohol. S/S includes ataxia, nystagmus, and seizures. Treat with IVFs, 5-10% ethanol infusion or fomepizole (Antizol), administer dextrose. Folic acid may prevent retinal toxicity in methanol toxicity.

- **Cannabis** – exposure to edibles increases risk, treatment is supportive.
- **Sympathomimetics** (cocaine, methamphetamine, ecstasy, bath salts) – S/S include altered mental status, tachycardia, hyperthermia, and seizures. Treatment includes cooling, benzodiazepines, sodium bicarbonate, and benzodiazepines.

- **Communicable Infections** (Refer to Chapter 8 in 6th edition ENPC)
  - **Meningitis** – S/S in infants: irritability, inconsolability, shrill cry, bulging fontanelle. S/S in children: fever, HA nuchal rigidity, opisthotonos, seizures, photophobia, Kernig's and Brudzinski's sign. DX: septic workup, lumbar puncture (side-lying position, oxygen during procedure, monitor respirations). TX: Isolation is priority, fluid boluses, vasopressors, antibiotics.
  - **Influenza** – prevent with vaccine yearly > 6 months. Avoid aspirin due to risk of Reye's syndrome. Teach caregivers thorough hand washing.
  - **Measles** (Rubeola) – S/S: the 3 C's – cough, coryza, and conjunctivitis, Koplik spots – blue-white spots on bright red buccal mucosa, maculopapular rash from hairline to face and downward. Incubation period is 7-14 days.
  - **Mumps (Parotitis)** – incubation 12-25 days. S/S: myalgias, swelling of the parotid and salivary glands, orchitis may cause sterility in males.
  - **Diphtheria** – grey pseudomembranous coating in back of throat. Incubation period is 1 to 8 days.
  - **Pertussis** – violent paroxysmal spasms of coughing, highly contagious through droplets. Incubation is 7 to 10 days.
  - **Mononucleosis** "kissing disease" – S/S: appear 4-6 weeks after infection, including extreme fatigue, fever, sore throat, swollen lymph nodes. TX: supportive care, avoid contact sports due to increased risk of splenic rupture.

Communicable Infections

- **Measles** (Rubeola) – 3 C's (conjunctivitis, coryza, cough) and Koplik spots. Standard and airborne isolation.
- **Mumps** – Salivary and parotid gland swelling, risk of orchitis. Standard and droplet precautions.
- **Pertussis** – Unremitting paroxysmal bursts of coughing. Standard and droplet precautions.
- **Diphtheria** – Thick, gray pseudomembranous coating on tonsils and pharynx. Standard and droplet precautions.

Multi-System Considerations (12 Exam Questions)

- **Submersion injury (Near-drowning)**
    - Risk: lack of supervision, inability to swim, alcohol or drug intoxication in adolescents, history of seizures or cardiac prolonged QT. Infants experience submersion more in bathtubs, children 1-4 are more likely to experience submersion in pools.
    - Potential spinal cord injury in diving incidents.
    - S/S: dyspnea, crackles, pink, frothy sputum.
    - TX: ABC's, warm the patient if severely hypothermic, NIPPV or endotracheal intubation with PEEP, insert gastric tube to decompress the stomach and minimize the risk of aspiration.
- **Sepsis**
    - Early S/S: – fever, tachycardia, **bounding pulses, flash capillary refill (< 1 second)**.
    - Late S/S: hypothermia, weak pulses, delayed capillary refill, hypotension.
    - DX: CBC and lactate.
    - TX: Isotonic crystalloid bolus of **10 to 20 mL/kg** up to 40 to 60 mL/kg over the first hour. Infuse epinephrine or norepinephrine, and antibiotics within 1 hour of ED arrival.
- **Anaphylaxis** – an overwhelming allergic reaction.
    - S/S: respiratory distress, hives, flushing, airway swelling, stridor, urticaria, wheezing, vomiting, and diarrhea.
    - TX: priority is **Epinephrine IM** in lateral thigh (**vastus lateralis**), inhaled albuterol, histamine blockers for urticaria and nausea/vomiting (diphenhydramine, famotidine), steroids.
- **Post-resuscitation (ROSC)** (PALS Chapter 13)
    - Maximize oxygenation and ventilation.
        - Maintain oxygen saturation at **94-99%**.
        - Monitor continuous waveform $ETCO_2$ capnography and keep at **35-45 mm Hg**.
        - Insert a gastric tube to relieve gastric inflation.
        - Avoid hyperventilation.
    - Restore preload with 10 to 20 mL/kg boluses of isotonic crystalloids.
    - Infuse epinephrine or norepinephrine for hypotensive shock.
    - Monitor glucose.
    - Control agitation with benzodiazepines, and control pain with analgesics like fentanyl, to hemodynamic stability.
    - Consider neuromuscular agents like vecuronium or rocuronium.
    - Consider targeted temperature management at 32 to 37 degrees Celsius initially, avoid shivering.
    - Maintenance fluid calculation by **4-2-1 method**.
        - < 10 kg – 4 mL/kg/hour
        - 10 to 20 kg – 40 mL/hour + 2 mL/kg/hour for each kg between 10 and 20 kg
        - > 20 kg – 60 mL/kg/hour + 1 mL/kg/hour for each kg above 20 kg
    - Manage increased intracranial pressure (ICP).
        - Elevate the head of bed to 30 degrees, keep head midline.
        - Administer mannitol or hypertonic saline.
    - Treat seizures aggressively.
- **Procedural sedation**
    - Obtain vital signs every 5 minutes.
    - Have suction equipment and intubation supplies at the bedside, pulse oximetry and continuous waveform ET CO_2 capnography.
    - Have reversal agents at the bedside.
    - Sedation discharge criteria Table 3-9

Professional Issues (12 Exam Questions)

- **Types of consent**
    - Implied – allows appropriate treatment in an emergency.
    - Express – written or oral agreement to testing and treatment.
    - Informed – full understanding of risks and benefits of proposed treatment.
    - Involuntary – invoked in a case of psychiatric, suicidal, or intoxicated patients.
- **Forensic evidence preservation**
    - Patient care takes precedence over forensic evidence collection.
    - Safeguard evidentiary materials by following chain of custody.
    - Avoid cutting through stains or holes in clothing.
    - Place clothing in separate clean paper bags to avoid condensation and degradation of evidence.
    - Document using verbatim, exact words even if vulgar terms are used. Do not document "patient alleges" or "claims", document "patient states" or "patient reports".
- **EMTALA** (Emergency Medical Treatment And Labor Act) **Standards**
    - Provide appropriate medical screening exam to determine the severity of the condition. (Nurse triage is not a medical screening exam).
    - Stabilize the patient within the capability of the hospital.
    - Ensure safe and medically necessary transfers of patients between facilities. Transfer the patient with appropriate personnel, equipment, and mode of transportation.
- **Workplace violence**
    - Nurses should make personal safety a priority. Never wear a stethoscope around your neck.
    - Nurses should deescalate themselves prior to de-escalation of aggressive individual.
    - Keep an exit for yourself.
    - Delay patient care until the risk of violence has decreased.
    - Report an assault to local law enforcement.
- **Active shooter**
    - Run away from the gunfire. Hide if you are unable to run away. Fight if you are cornered.
    - Secure the location, barricade the doors. Preserve life and fight if necessary.
- **Drug diversion –** install systems to guard against diversion, monitor high-risk areas, train staff on recognition, and promote "see something, say something." Report any suspicion to a supervisor immediately.
- **Culture of safety (Just Culture)** – empower nurses to report near misses and errors.
- **Delegation** – a nurse may not delegate any task to unlicensed assistive personnel that involves nursing judgement or critical decision-making.
- **Discharge planning education**
    - Ask Me 3 - What is my main problem? What do I need to do? Why is it important for me to do this?
    - Teach Back
        - Sit at eye level and make eye contact.
        - Use clear, plain language. Example: "Can you show me…?"
- **Patient safety** – weigh children in **kilograms only** to avoid double-dosing.
- **Person-first language** – less stigmatizing and reduces bias. State "a child experiencing homelessness" instead a "homeless person" or a "person with addiction" not "an addict".
- **Transgender patient** – inquire "how can I best address you?"
- **Trauma-informed care** – avoid retraumatizing the patient by ensuring safety and practicing family-centered care. Ask, "what happened to you?", not "What is wrong with you?"
- According to the National Highway Traffic Safety Administration (NHTSA), 50% of child safety seats are installed or used incorrectly. Children should sit in the **back seat for safety** until at least age 12.

- **Injury prevention purpose** (TNCC pg. 4)
  - Primary – prevention of the occurrence of the injury.
  - Secondary – reduction of the severity of the injury that has already occurred.
  - Tertiary – improvement of the outcome related to the traumatic injury.

PDB Nurse Education, LLC CPEN Primary References

- American Heart Association, *Manual of Pediatric Advanced Life Support* (PALS), 2020.
- Emergency Nurses Association. *Emergency Nurses Pediatric Course Provider Manual*, 5th edition, 2020.
- Emergency Nurses Association. *Emergency Nurses Pediatric Course Provider Manual*, 6th edition, 2023.
- Emergency Nurses Association. *Emergency Severity Index Handbook*, 5th edition, 2023.
- Emergency Nurses Association. *Sheehy's Emergency Nursing: Principles and Practice*, 7th ed., 2020.
- Emergency Nurses Association. *Sheehy's Manual of Emergency Care*, 8th ed., 2024.
- Emergency Nurses Association. *Trauma Nursing Core Curriculum, 8th* ed., 2019.
- Emergency Nurses Association. *Trauma Nursing Core Curriculum, 9th* ed., 2024.

This Study Guide is registered with the Board of Certification for Emergency Nursing (BCEN®); however, they do not endorse any resource or have a proprietary relationship with any publishing company.

CPEN Triage Process (20 Exam Questions, 27 Samples)

1. What are the three components of the pediatric assessment triangle (PAT)?
    a. Airway status, work of breathing, circulation to skin
    b. Appearance, work of breathing, circulation to skin
    c. Appearance, work of breathing, obvious bleeding
    d. Airway status, work of breathing, obvious bleeding

    B – The components of the PAT are general **A**ppearance, work of **B**reathing, **C**irculation. PAT is a "quick look" to determine if a child is "sick", "sicker", or "sickest". (ENPC pgs. 48-49 and PALS pg. 40)

2. Which mnemonic is useful for assessing general appearance when using the pediatric assessment triangle (PAT)?
    a. APGAR
    b. MUDPILES
    c. TICLS
    d. 5 P's

    C – TICLS is the mnemonic used to remember what to assess during the across-the-room initial assessment regarding a patient's general appearance. **T**one: moving vs. limp and flaccid, **I**nteractiveness: does the child appear interested in his/her surroundings, **C**onsolability: is the child easily comforted, **L**ook/gaze: is the child alert or staring into space, **S**peech/cry: strong or weak? (ENPC pg. 49 and PALS pg. 40)

3. A mother brings her 7-year-old daughter to the ED complaining of ear pain for 3 days. Your across-the-room assessment reveals an alert child who is playing with her doll, respirations even and unlabored, and skin is pink. How would you categorize this child?
    a. Not sick
    b. Sick
    c. Sicker
    d. Sickest

    B – There is **no** disruption to any component of the PAT, but the **caregiver is concerned** enough to seek medical care. This child falls into the "sick" category (ENPC pg. 50)

4. An 8-year-old patient is brought to the ED by his mother complaining of asthma exacerbation. Your across-the-room assessment reveals an alert child who is interacting appropriately with his mother, audible wheezing with accessory muscle use, and pink skin. How would you categorize this patient?
    a. Not sick
    b. Sick
    c. Sicker
    d. Sickest

    C – This patient is considered "sicker" because **one** component of the PAT (work of breathing) is abnormal. (ENPC pg. 50)

5. A 3-year-old child is brought to the ED via EMS. Across-the-room assessment reveals a lethargic child with retractions and wheezing, with pink skin. How would you categorize this patient?
    a. Not sick
    b. Sick
    c. Sicker
    d. Sickest

    D – There is an abnormality to **two** components of the PAT (appearance and breathing), making this patient fall into the sickest category. (ENPC pg. 50)

6. What is the leading cause of death in children between the ages of 0 to 19?
    a. Suffocation
    b. Intentional injury
    c. Unintentional injury
    d. Sports-related injury

C – The leading cause of death in children between the ages of 0 and 19 is **unintentional injury**, such as motor vehicle collisions, firearms, drowning, and falls. The major cause of death in infants is suffocation. Caregiver education should include information on prevention of unintentional injury. (ENPC pg. 129)

7. A patient assigned female sex at birth complains of abdominal pain. Her last menstrual period is reported as 8 weeks ago. Her heart rate is 124 beats/minute and blood pressure is 88/54 mm Hg. The triage nurse suspects a ruptured ectopic pregnancy so assigns the patient which triage level utilizing Emergency Severity Index (ESI) Triage?
    a. ESI level 1
    b. ESI level 2
    c. ESI level 3
    d. ESI level 4

B – This patient will be uptriaged to ESI level 2 based on her vital signs and suspicion of bleeding. (ENPC pgs. 54-56 and ESI Triage Handbook, 5th edition.)

8. Relying on the Pediatric Assessment Triangle, the emergency nurse knows which of the following would be the most concerning when assessing a 9-month-old infant?
    a. Temperature of 100.2 F (37.9 C).
    b. Pale skin with mottling to extremities.
    c. Even, unlabored respirations at 38 breaths/minute.
    d. Three episodes of semi-formed stools in the last 24 hours.

B - **Pale skin** is noticed in appearance and circulation in PAT. You would not obtain a temperature in PAT. The other indicators are normal in a 9-month-old. (ENPC pgs. 48-49)

9. Which patient should be triaged first?
    a. 10-year-old with a history of asthma, with minor wheezing.
    b. 12-year-old with blunt abdominal trauma who is pale and has a heart rate of 150.
    c. 18-month-old who now has purulent drainage from the ear.
    d. 15-year-old who went hiking in the woods last week and now has a rash on arms and hands.

B - The patient with blunt abdominal trauma and **signs of shock** is the priority. The other complaints are less urgent. (ENPC pgs. 48-49)

10. Four patients with complaints of headaches present to your triage desk within minutes. You consider which of the following complaints the most emergent?
    a. 16-year-old with a throbbing headache asking, "can you turn off the lights?"
    b. 14-year-old with sudden onset of a severe headache who has vomited twice in the last 30 minutes.
    c. 8-year-old with a headache and rhinitis.
    d. 4-year-old with redness and swelling on her forehead after falling one step.

B – Sudden onset of severe headache with **vomiting** may be symptoms of increased intracranial pressure. (ENPC pgs. 48-49)

11. Applying the principles of the Pediatric Assessment Triangle, which of the following patients should be triaged first?
    a. A 3-year-old who is lying in his mother's lap; has dry, cracked lips; and is pale.
    b. A 2-year-old who is crying intermittently while throwing her toy onto the floor.
    c. A child sitting in a chair with an occasional nonproductive cough and red cheeks.
    d. An 18-month-old with red cheeks and a sweaty forehead who is bundled up in several blankets.

A - Pale skin with dry cracked lips are signs of **dehydration** noticed in Appearance and Circulation in PAT. Crying intermittently, a nonproductive cough, and red cheeks are less urgent signs/symptoms. (ENPC pgs. 48-49)

12. Based on the appearance of the following patients, which one should be brought back first?
    a. A 2-year-old who swallowed a quarter, with clear breath sounds and playing with his toys.
    b. A 10-year-old with a history of asthma who has scattered expiratory wheezing and an O_2 sat of 95%, who ran out of his inhaler.
    c. A 3-year-old who is tachypneic, drooling, and appears anxious.
    d. A 9-year-old male sent to the ED by the school nurse for abdominal pain who is bent over holding his abdomen.

C – Tachypnea, **drooling**, and anxiety are signs/symptoms of a partially obstructed airway. Airway obstruction is more emergent than mild asthma exacerbation, stable foreign body ingestion, or possible appendicitis. (ENPC pgs. 48-49)

13. Which of these patients is the priority?
    a. A patient with sickle cell crisis complaining of chest pain.
    b. A patient who is postictal after experiencing a febrile seizure.
    c. A child with a wrist deformity after falling on the playground.
    d. A child with hemophilia who has a cough.

A – Acute chest syndrome is the number one cause of death in patients with sickle cell disease. S/S: chest pain, fever, cough, shortness of breath. DX: chest x-ray revealing pulmonary infiltrates. TX: IV hydration, antibiotics, and pain management. (ENPC pgs. 48-49)

14. Which of the following patients requires immediate intervention?
    a. A 5-year-old child with a history of asthma who has a fever.
    b. An infant who has been crying for 3 hours straight and his father noticed that his middle toe is turning dark purple.
    c. A 7-year-old who fell at the playground and complains of wrist pain.
    d. A 10-year-old with a history of epilepsy who complains of a headache.

B – A hair tourniquet can be a reason that an infant is fussy that requires immediate intervention to restore circulation to the limb (toe, finger, penis, clitoris). If an infant or toddler is fussy/crying for no apparent reason, it is important to complete a full head-to-toe assessment to ensure that there is not a hair tourniquet present. Other possible causes of crying infant can be explored using the **"AH IF IT CRIES"** mnemonic (ENPC pg. 61)

AH! IF IT CRIESS

- Anger
- Hunger
- Infection
- Fear/Frustration
- Increased ICP
- Trauma/Testicular Torsion
- Cardiac issues
- Reflux/Reaction
- Immunizations/Insect bites
- Eye (corneal abrasion, FB)
- Surgical (intussusception, volvulus, hernia)
- Strangulation (hair tourniquet)

ENPC 6th edition pg. 61

15. Which of the following patients presenting to the pediatric emergency department should be assigned a bed first?
    a. A 3-year-old with a history of cystic fibrosis complaining of nausea and vomiting for two days; across the room assessment reveals pink skin, unlabored breathing, and patient appears tired, resting in mother's arms.
    b. A 5-year-old patient with a history of complaining of abdominal pain and constipation for five days; across the room assessment reveals pink skin, unlabored breathing, and patient appears tired, resting in mother's arms.
    c. A 4-year-old patient with a history of asthma complaining of fever and ear pain; across the room assessment reveals pink skin, unlabored breathing, and patient appears tired, resting in mother's arms.
    d. A 2-month-old patient with Hirschsprung's Disease, with fever, diarrhea, and a distended abdomen.

D – Hirschsprung-associated enterocolitis is also known as aganglionic megacolon and is a congenital disorder that occurs when there is no nerve innervation to create peristalsis in the distant bowel. Most cases are diagnosed during the neonatal period and are characterized by no passing of meconium within the first 2 days of life, abdominal distention, feeding intolerance, and bilious emesis. Treatment often requires surgical intervention (ENPC pgs. 176-177)

16. Which of the following patients is the highest priority?
    a. A patient with asthma complaining of productive cough and fever.
    b. A patient with sickle cell disease complaining of fever.
    c. A patient with autism spectrum disorder with a laceration of the arm.
    d. A patient with epilepsy complaining of a fever and sore throat.

B - Fever in patients with sickle cell disease is considered a medical emergency due to their compromised immune function. (ENPC pgs. 282-283)

17. A 2-year-old without airway compromise swallowed an alkaline button battery. Vital signs are within normal limits. The correct ESI priority is:
    a. ESI level 1
    b. ESI level 2
    c. ESI level 3
    d. ESI level 4

B – ESI level 2. Esophageal button battery ingestion has a high risk of complications so is extremely time sensitive. (ENPC pgs. 54-56 and ESI Triage Handbook 5th edition)

18. "I just turned my back for a minute," cried the mother of a 4-year-old. The child was pulled out of the family pool by a neighbor who immediately administered mouth-to-mouth resuscitation. The child is now breathing spontaneously but continues to be unresponsive. On arrival to the ED vital signs are HR=126, RR=28, BP=80/64, SpO_2=96% on a non-rebreather. The correct ESI priority is:
    a. ESI level 1
    b. ESI level 2
    c. ESI level 3
    d. ESI level 4

A - ESI triage level 1 due to unresponsiveness, regardless of vital signs. (ENPC pgs. 54-56 and ESI Triage 5th edition)

19. A mom brings in her 14-year-old requesting he be checked. He has a severe shellfish allergy and mistakenly ate a dip that contained shrimp. He immediately felt his throat start to close so used his Epi Pen. He tells you he feels okay. No wheezes or rash are noted. VS: HR=108, RR=20, BP=126/74, SpO_2 96%. The correct ESI priority is:
    a. ESI level 1
    b. ESI level 2
    c. ESI level 3
    d. ESI level 4

B - ESI triage level **2** due to high risk of airway obstruction from anaphylaxis. (ENPC pgs. 54-56 and ESI Triage Handbook 5th edition)

20. A 15-year-old handcuffed male is escorted into the ED by the police. The parents called 911 because their son was out of control, threatening to kill the family. He answers your questions appropriately, has no past medical history, and is taking no medications. Vital signs are within normal limits. The correct ESI priority is:
    a. ESI level 1
    b. ESI level 2
    c. ESI level 3
    d. ESI level 4

B - ESI triage level 2 due to high risk for situation/safety. (ENPC pgs. 54-65 and ESI Triage 5th edition)

21. What is the most accurate way to determine a pediatric patient's weight in triage?
    a. Use a scale that measures in kilograms.
    b. Use a scale that measures in pounds.
    c. Use a colored-coded, length-based measuring tape.
    d. Ask the caregiver what their most recent weight was.

A – Weigh the patient on a scale that measures in **kilograms**. Lock the scale in kilograms to avoid accidentally measuring in pounds and documenting as kilograms. Avoid calculating pounds to kilograms due to the risk of error and double dosing the child. (ENPC pg. 33)

22. Patients with suspected testicular or ovarian torsion should be triaged as which ESI triage level?
    a. ESI level 1
    b. ESI level 2
    c. ESI level 3
    d. ESI level 4

B – ESI level 2. Torsion is a time-sensitive clinical situation capable of producing permanent organ loss. (ENPC pgs. 54-56 and ESI Triage Handbook 5th edition)

23. The best approach to assessing suicide risk in an adolescent with a history of depression would be to:
    a. Ask the parents.
    b. Assume suicide risk based on the history of depression.
    c. Ask the patient directly if they have thoughts of hurting themselves.
    d. Let the ED physician or mental health counselor ask the patient.

C - Ask the patient directly in the initial triage assessment for proper placement in the department. Increase risk of suicide if previous attempts, family history of suicide, having a plan to commit suicide. (ENPC pg. 243)

24. During a disaster, the pediatric emergency nurse is assigned to the cold zone where he knows his duties are best described as providing:
    a. Basic life support only until decontamination has occurred.
    b. Warming measures for hypothermic patients.
    c. Complete nursing care as required.
    d. Scrubbing with soap and water for a minimum of 5 minutes.

C - Complete care is given in the cold zone. Only Hazmat trained personnel go into the hot zone, where only life-saving treatment is performed. Decontamination occurs in the warm zone. Decontamination tents are set up so patient flow is opposite of wind direction.

25. A tornado just struck a large school, and you are triaging in the community. A child is found unresponsive, with agonal respirations and a weak pulse. Using the Jump START triage, what triage category should this child fall into?
    a. Red
    b. Green
    c. Yellow
    d. Black

A - Red due to agonal respirations. START triage is based on if the patient is ambulatory "Green", then RPM - respiration, perfusion (capillary refill), and mental status. "Red" are the priority to get to treatment immediately, "Yellow" is delayed, "Black" is expectant to die. (ENPC pg. 58)

26. Using the JumpSTART triage, which triage category assignment would the nurse give to a 5-year-old who is lying on the ground, alert and crying with spontaneous respirations of 36 breaths/minute and normal peripheral pulses?
    a. Red
    b. Green
    c. Yellow
    d. Black

C- Yellow, since the child is non-ambulatory but everything else is within normal limits per RPM (respirations between 15 and 45, capillary refill < 2 seconds, able to follow commands). (ENPC pg. 58)

27. During a mass casualty incident (MCI) there are multiple pediatric patients arriving to the ED and you are applying Jump START criteria to triage the patients. You are triaging a 5-year-old patient who is unconscious, pale, and limp. She is not breathing, even after opening her airway. She has a palpable pulse. What is your next action?
    a. Categorize as deceased/expectant and move on to the next patient.
    b. Provide 5 rescue breaths and reassess breathing.
    c. Begin chest compressions and rescue breathing.
    d. Categorize the patient as immediate and begin rescue breathing.

B – The difference between **START** and **JumpSTART** disaster triage criteria is that **5 rescue breaths** are to be provided to a pediatric patient who is not breathing but has a palpable pulse, and breathing is to be reassessed prior to categorizing the patient as dead/dying. If this patient begins breathing on her own after 5 rescue breaths, they would be categorized as immediate (Red). (ENPC pg. 58)

CPEN Assessment (25 Exam Questions, 25 Samples)

1. Stridor during the inspiratory phase of the respiratory cycle is heard in which respiratory disorder?
   a. Upper airway obstruction
   b. Lower airway obstruction
   c. Lung tissue disease
   d. Disordered control of breathing

   A - Stridor (typically inspiratory), along with a barking cough is heard in **upper airway obstruction**. Wheezing (typically expiratory) is heard in lower airway obstruction. Grunting and crackles are audible in lung tissue disease. (PALS pgs. 119 and 122)

2. What is the minimum acceptable systolic blood pressure for a 2-year-old?
   a. 54 mm hg
   b. 64 mm hg
   c. 74 mm hg
   d. 84 mm hg

   C – 74 mm Hg. Hypotension is defined as SBP < 60 mm Hg for neonate, < 70 for 1-year-old, and < 70 + (2 x age in years) for 1-10. For children > 10 years of age, < 90 mm Hg is defined as hypotension. (ENPC pgs. 34 and 99, PALS pg. 58)

3. Young children have a natural anatomical condition which causes:
   a. Neck extension when lying on a flat surface.
   b. Back extension when lying on a flat surface.
   c. Neck flexion when lying on a flat surface.
   d. Back flexion when lying on a flat surface.

   C – Neck flexion. Infants and young children have a proportionally larger occiput increasing the potential for airway obstruction when they are in a supine position due to hyperflexion of the neck. Place padding under the shoulders and upper torso to provide a neutral position. (ENPC pg. 71, PALS pg. 147)

4. When examining a 2-year-old, keep all the following in mind, **EXCEPT**:
   a. Evaluate uninjured and painless parts first.
   b. They may exhibit separation anxiety.
   c. Toddlers should be examined away from the caregiver.
   d. Parents can be helpful with examining the child.

   C is an **incorrect** statement. **Parents are a valuable source** of information and guidance, and 2-year-olds need caregivers close by. Always examine painful areas last. (ENPC pg. 30)

5. The best way to communicate information to preschool children is to use:
   a. Detailed anatomical models to better illustrate procedures.
   b. Word games like "taking your pulse" or "shooting an X-ray".
   c. Simple, concrete terminology.
   d. Cooperative decision-making processes such as asking questions like "Can we start an IV now?"

   C – Use **simple, concrete terminology**, and play therapy when communicating with preschoolers. (ENPC pgs. 30-32)

6. You hear stridor in a 1-year-old in respiratory distress. This represents:
   a. Rapid Kussmaul's breathing associated with diabetic ketoacidosis (DKA).
   b. A high-pitched sound heard on inspiration associated with upper respiratory obstruction.
   c. A whistling sound produced by air moving through narrow airways.
   d. A crackling sound heard in pulmonary edema.

B - **Stridor** (high-pitched sound heard on inspiration) is associated with upper airway disorders, like croup, anaphylaxis, or epiglottitis. (ENPC pg. 49, PALS pg. 50)

7. When telling a preschooler about an upcoming procedure, it is most appropriate to:
   a. Tell them hours in advance.
   b. Tell them it will not hurt.
   c. Tell them immediately prior to the procedure.
   d. Do not tell them anything, just hold them down and do it quickly.

C - Tell the preschooler **immediately prior** to procedure and be honest about pain. Say "take a nap", not "put you to sleep."

8. Appropriate urine output for a 10 kg child is:
   a. 0.1 mL/hour
   b. 10-20 mL/hour
   c. 30 mL/kg
   d. 100 mL/hour

B - **10-20 mL/hour** for a 10 kg child (1-2 ml/kg/hour) Urine output < 1 mL/kg/hour indicates poor end-organ perfusion. (ENPC pg. 79 and PALS pg. 53)

9. The parent of a 2-year-old is frustrated with her child's behavior. He throws temper tantrums and says "NO" to everything. The nurse explains this is a normal response as 2-year-olds try to:
   a. Increase their independence.
   b. Gratify their oral fixation.
   c. Complete everything they start.
   d. Establish trust.

A – The toddler is most concerned with achieving some sense of **independence**.

10. The nurse is positioning an infant for a procedure. Which of the following indicators is a reliable sign that the infant is in pain?
    a. Facial expressions
    b. Squirming
    c. Crying
    d. Body rigidity

A - **Facial expressions** like grimacing and chin quivering are signs of pain. (ENPC pg. 40)

11. Which of the following is the most important source of information when caring for a child with a complex medical history in the ED?
    a. The child's previous medical records.
    b. The child's family or primary caregiver.
    c. The ED team's knowledge of the child's illness.
    d. Published reference sources.

B - The child's family or **primary caregiver is the expert** and can give insight into the child's baseline behaviors, neurologic status, abilities, and overall health, so that concerning deviations from baselines can be identified. (ENPC pg. 20)

12. Which of the following are the most ominous signs of respiratory failure?
    a. Tachypnea and tachycardia
    b. Tachypnea and bradycardia
    c. Bradypnea and tachycardia
    d. Bradypnea and bradycardia

D - **Bradypnea and bradycardia** are late (ominous) signs related to hypoxia and may indicate impending arrest. Tachypnea and tachycardia are signs of respiratory distress. (ENPC pg. 118 and PALS pg. 122)

13. The nursing assessment and history of a child of suspected maltreatment should include which of the following?
    a. Expressing concern to the caregivers about the lack of appropriate parenting skills.
    b. Asking the caregivers to wait to explain how the injury occurred until law enforcement arrives.
    c. Documenting any relevant verbal statements from the caregivers in quotes.
    d. Promising the child that you will not tell anyone what they say.

C - **Document the questions asked, the responses verbatim**, and the emotional reactions observed during the interview. (ENPC pg. 264)

14. Which of the following pain assessment scales is most appropriate to use for a 2-year-old?
    a. Numeric scale (0-10).
    b. Revised FLACC scale (face, legs, activity, cry, consolability).
    c. FACES pain rating scale.
    d. NIPS scale.

B – The **revised FLACC** scale is recommended for preverbal children and the cognitively impaired child. The FACES scale is recommended for children 4-12 years of age and the numeric scale for approximately 8 years of age. NIPS scale is recommended for infants up to one year of age. (ENPC pg. 40)

15. You are triaging an 11-year-old patient who presents to the ED for vomiting. The patient's mother states that the patient has special needs and that he is nonverbal and uses a wheelchair. All the following are true about caring for children with special needs**, EXCEPT**:
    a. Include the parents in your assessment of the patient, they are often experts in understanding their child's condition and unique baseline status.
    b. Always use the FACES pain scale for a patient who is nonverbal.
    c. Use "people first" language when speaking about the patient, ex: child with autism, not an autistic child.
    d. Avoid using negative descriptions such as "suffers from" or "afflicted with".

B – The **revised FLACC** (Face, Legs, Activity, Cry, Consolability) scale not FACES, is appropriate for use with patients with cognitive impairment. The other options are correct. (ENPC pgs. 40 and 279-280)

16. A 15-year-old girl complaining of abdominal pain is brought to the ED by her father. The following considerations should be followed with a child this age, **EXCEPT**:
    a. Speak to the child in a respectful manner, as if speaking to an adult.
    b. When speaking to the caregiver, include the child.
    c. Tell the father you suspect the child is sexually active.
    d. Obtain the sexual history without the caregiver in the room.

C – Protect the **adolescent's privacy**, do not tell the father his child is sexually active. (ENPC pg. 33)

17. Wheezing during the inspiratory phase of the respiratory cycle is heard in which respiratory disorder?
    a. Upper airway obstruction
    b. Lower airway obstruction
    c. Lung tissue disease
    d. Disordered control of breathing

B - Wheezing (typically expiratory) is heard in lower airway obstruction. Grunting and crackles are audible in lung tissue disease. (PALS pgs. 120 and 122)

18. How do you classify a toddler who recognizes their caregivers but does not respond to requests of the healthcare team?
    a. Alert
    b. Verbal
    c. Pain
    d. Unresponsive

A – **Alert**. An alert older infant or toddler will recognize their caregivers, be cautious of strangers, and may not respond to requests of the healthcare team. (TNCC pg. 275)

19. Which of the following parameters is NOT assessed when calculating a Glasgow Coma Scale (GCS)?
    a. Eye opening
    b. Verbal response
    c. Motor response
    d. Pupillary response

D – **Pupillary response** is not a component of the Glasgow Coma Scale (GCS). A GCS score of 13-15 is associated with mild traumatic brain injury, a score of 9-12 is associated with moderate brain injury, and a score of less than 9 is associated with severe brain injury. (ENPC pgs. 73-74)

20. Which burn is not as suspicious for intentional injury?
    a. Grouped circular burns on the back.
    b. Sock-like burns to bilateral lower extremities, without splash marks.
    c. Buttock burn with donut hole skin sparing.
    d. A burn in a geometric pattern.

A – **Grouped circular burns** or ecchymoses on the back may be caused by **cupping** to "draw out" the ailment. Sock-like or glove-like burns with sharp demarcated margins, burns where skin folds are spared, and patterned burns are more likely inflicted burns. (ENPC pgs. 259-262)

21. Which of the following statements is **CORRECT** regarding infant growth?
    a. An infant's weight should approximately double by three months of age.
    b. An infant's weight should approximately double by six months of age.
    c. An infant's weight should approximately triple by six months of age.
    d. An infant's weight should approximately triple by nine months of age.

B – An infant's weight should **double by six months of age**, and triple by twelve months of age. Infancy is a period of rapid growth. Toddlers gain < or = to 5 pounds/year. (Sheehy pg. 454)

22. Which of the following statements is **CORRECT** regarding infant motor development?
    a. An infant should be able to lift their head when prone by 3 months.
    b. An infant should be able to turn over when prone by 3 months.
    c. An infant should be able to sit unsupported by 6 months.
    d. An infant should be able to stand by 9 months.

B – Generally, an infant should be able to lift their head when prone by 3 months, turn over by 6 months, sit unsupported by 9 months, and stand by 12 months of age. (ENPC pg. 30 and Sheehy pg. 454)

23. Erikson's autonomy versus shame and doubt occurs in which psychosocial developmental stage of the life cycle?
    a. Infancy
    b. Toddler
    c. Preschool
    d. School-age

B – Toddlers experience autonomy versus shame and doubt. Infants experience trust versus mistrust. Preschoolers experience initiative versus guilt. School-age children experience industry versus inferiority. (ENPC pg. 30 and Sheehy pg. 454)

24. Calloused hands and tooth erosion is more commonly assessed in which psychological disorder?
    a. Bulimia nervosa
    b. Anorexia nervosa
    c. Post-traumatic stress disorder
    d. Attention deficit hyperactivity disorder.

A – Self-induced vomiting related to bulimia nervosa results in calloused hands and tooth erosion. (ENPC pg. 248)

25. Which of the following statements regarding ketamine is **INCORRECT**?
    a. Ketamine can be safely administered intranasally.
    b. Ketamine provides sedation, analgesia, and amnesia.
    c. Emergence reaction is common.
    d. The half-life of ketamine is 2.5 hours.

    C – **Emergence reaction (agitation) is uncommon** with Ketamine administration. Ketamine can be administered intranasally, intramuscularly, and intravenously, with a half-life of 2.5 hours. (ENPC pg. 41)

System-Focused Emergencies (56 Exam Questions, 76 Samples)

1. A 1-month-old infant arrives at the ED with a heart rate of 20. The nurse realizes that bradycardias in infants are usually first treated with:
    a. Epinephrine
    b. Atropine
    c. Chest compressions
    d. Bag-mask ventilations with 100% oxygen

    D - Most bradycardias in infants are due to respiratory distress/arrest so the priority is to **assist ventilation with bag-mask ventilations**. (PALS pg. 244)

2. You are caring for a 10-year-old who was brought in by EMS after being involved in an MVC. The patient complains of chest pain and shortness of breath. Vital signs are HR 160, BP 75/32, RR 35 and labored. Your assessment reveals distended neck veins and absent breath sounds on the right side. What should be done for this patient first?
    a. Obtain a chest x-ray.
    b. Needle decompression of right chest.
    c. Needle decompression of left chest.
    d. Initiate IV and administer 20mL/kg of isotonic fluid.

    B – This patient is exhibiting signs and symptoms of a tension pneumothorax on the right side. This patient requires **immediate needle decompression** on the affected side followed by chest tube insertion. Intervention should be immediate without waiting for chest x-ray. (ENPC pg. 134 and PALS pg. 220)

3. EMS brings in a child in cardiac arrest with compressions and bag-mask ventilations in progress. The practitioner intubates the patient and confirms placement, but it is difficult to ventilate the patient. Breath sounds are auscultated in all lung fields. What priority nursing intervention may improve ventilation?
    a. Attaching to a ventilator and add PEEP.
    b. Increasing the rate of ventilation.
    c. Increasing the oxygen concentration to 100%.
    d. Inserting a gastric tube.

    D - **Inserting a gastric tube** to decompress stomach since ventilations cause gastric distension. Gastric distention impairs adequate ventilation by impeding downward movement of the diaphragm. (ENPC pg. 76)

4. You are treating a child in cardiac arrest. CPR is initiated, and the cardiac monitor reveals ventricular fibrillation (VF). Which of the following should be performed immediately?
    a. Establish IO access and administer epinephrine.
    b. Perform synchronized cardioversion at 0.5-1.0 j/kg.
    c. Defibrillate at 2-4 j/kg.
    d. Intubate the patient.

C - CPR and defibrillation are the priorities in VF, along with finding the cause of the arrest and administering IV/IO epinephrine. (PALS pg. 90 and ENPC pg. 113)

5. A 7-year-old patient is brought in by his father stating that he was complaining of shortness of breath and diaphoretic. At the time of arrival, the patient is obtunded, with a heart rate of 200 on the monitor with narrow and regular QRS complex and a blood pressure of 85/43. What is the most appropriate next action?
    a. Defibrillate the patient at 2-4j/kg.
    b. Synchronized cardioversion at 0.5-1 j/kg.
    c. Administer adenosine 0.1mg/kg.
    d. Perform vagal maneuvers by having the child blow through a straw.

B – This patient is experiencing unstable SVT and requires **immediate synchronized cardioversion**. Adenosine administration and vagal maneuvers would be appropriate for a patient with stable SVT. Defibrillate a patient with pulseless shockable rhythms VT or VF. (PALS pg. 255)

6. A 5-day-old infant is brought to the emergency department for decreased feeding, tachypnea, cyanosis, and lethargy. If this patient is suspected to have a PDA-dependent lesion, which of the following medications do you expect to be ordered?
    a. High-flow oxygen
    b. Beta-2 Agonist
    c. Indomethacin/Ibuprofen
    d. Prostaglandin E1

D – Prostaglandin E1 (PGE1) should be initiated immediately if there is suspicion of a possible cardiac PDA-dependent lesion. Prostaglandin E1 helps maintain an open PDA. High-flow oxygen and indomethacin/ibuprofen are used to close a PDA which may worsen symptoms. The timing of these symptoms could align with closure of the PDA. (ENPC pg. 88 and PALS pg. 220)

7. What is the best way to monitor ventilation?
    a. Visually monitor rate, depth, and work of breathing.
    b. Monitor skin color.
    c. Monitor SaO_2
    d. Monitor $ETCO_2$ capnography.

D – $ETCO_2$ waveform capnography monitoring provides continuous information about ventilation. Normal values are 35-45mmHg. Changes can be detected much sooner with waveform capnography than with SaO_2 monitoring alone. (ENPC pg. 76)

8. A patient who presents with croup after chest x-ray reveals steeple sign. Which treatments does the pediatric emergency nurse expect to be ordered by the provider if the patient has stridor at rest?
    a. Dexamethasone and albuterol.
    b. Nasal suctioning and humidified oxygen.
    c. Nebulized epinephrine and dexamethasone.
    d. Antibiotics and prednisone.

C – Treat severe croup with **nebulized racemic epinephrine and dexamethasone**. (ENPC pg. 124 and PALS pgs. 128-129)

9. You are providing discharge teaching to a parent of a child diagnosed with croup. Which statement indicates that the parent requires additional education?
    a. I need to make sure that she is drinking plenty of fluids.
    b. I will come back if her condition worsens.
    c. I will make sure to keep her in a warm, dry environment.
    d. I will administer ibuprofen as needed for fever.

C – Do not keep the child in a warm, dry area. Discharge instructions for croup include taking the child into cool air, using a cool mist humidifier, taking the child into a steamy bathroom, encouraging oral hydration, administering antipyretics for fever, and returning for signs of respiratory distress, fatigue, and stridor at rest. (ENPC pg. 124)

10. You are triaging for a 3-year-old who presents with stridor, drooling, and fever. He is tripoding with an SaO_2 of 91% on room air. What is the appropriate next step for this patient?
    a. Take the patient out of the mother's arms and lay him flat on the bed to perform a thorough examination.
    b. Have the caregiver hold him while an ABG is obtained to ensure that he has adequate ventilation.
    c. Use a tongue depressor to better assess for enlarged, purulent tonsils.
    d. Let his caregiver hold him, administer blow-by oxygen, and arrange for airway assessment in the emergency department or operating room.

D – Stridor with drooling indicate possible epiglottitis. **Let the caregiver hold the child** and care for the patient in a non-stimulating environment. Avoid activities that will cause the patient to become anxious or cry. One-third of patients require intubation and are likely to become difficult airways. Airway assessment and intubation should be performed in the emergency department or operating room with a surgical airway prepared as backup. (ENPC pgs. 123-124)

11. The induction agent of choice for a decompensating patient presenting with asthma is:
    a. Ketamine
    b. Versed
    c. Etomidate
    d. Propofol

A – Ketamine is a hypnotic dissociative analgesic medication that is also a potent bronchodilator, which is appropriate for use in asthmatic patients prior to intubation. Use caution with increased secretions in airway as ketamine may increase secretions. Administer Atropine or Scopolamine to reduce secretions if needed. (ENPC pg. 122)

12. Which of the following is the **MOST** concerning triage assessment finding in a patient with an asthma exacerbation?
    a. Prolonged expiratory phase with wheezing.
    b. Absence of wheezing.
    c. A patient who can speak 2-3 words at a time.
    d. Increased wheezing after nebulizer treatment.

B – Absence of wheezing may indicate severe airway constriction and is an ominous sign. Increasing wheezing may be a result of opening airways if previously severely constricted. A prolonged expiratory phase with wheezing is a common finding in a patient with asthma exacerbation. (ENPC pg. 121 and PALS pgs. 132-133)

13. What test is used to assess the severity of an asthma exacerbation?
    a. Steeple sign on x-ray.
    b. Peak flow
    c. Thumbprint sign on x-ray.
    d. Infiltrates on chest x-ray.

B – Compare **peak flow measurement** to previous measurements for the child to determine severity of asthma exacerbation. Children older than 4-5 years old should be able to perform this test. Steeple sign is indicative of croup, and thumbprint sign on lateral neck x-ray is indicative of epiglottitis. A chest x-ray can be used to rule out pneumonia. (ENPC pg. 121 and PALS pgs. 132-133)

14. What treatments can the pediatric emergency nurse expect to be ordered for a patient presenting with asthma exacerbation?
    a. Albuterol, ipratropium, steroids, magnesium.
    b. Humidified oxygen, cool air, steamy bathroom.
    c. Albuterol, antibiotics, oxygen.
    d. Racemic epinephrine, steroids, albuterol.

A – Albuterol is an inhaled short-acting beta-agonist bronchodilator, **ipratropium** (Atrovent) is an inhaled anticholinergic, early **steroids** may reduce time in ED and hospital admissions. **IV magnesium sulfate**, or terbutaline may be used if the patient does not respond to standard therapy. IV or PO fluids can help loosen secretions and prevent mucus plugging. (ENPC pg. 121 and PALS pg. 133)

15. A 2-year-old patient is brought in by their mother. The mother states that the patient is unvaccinated and states that for the past week the patient has had a severe cough with a loud "whoop" on inspiration, followed by vomiting. What isolation precautions should be taken for this patient?
    a. Standard precautions only.
    b. Standard and contact precautions.
    c. Standard and droplet precautions.
    d. Standard and airborne precautions.

C – Droplet precautions should be initiated for pertussis, also known as "whooping cough." This is a reportable disease that should be reported to the CDC. Erythromycin is the antibiotic of choice. (ENPC pg. 124)

Isolation Precautions

Airborne Precautions

- Tuberculosis, Measles (Rubeola), Chickenpox (Varicella).
- Negative pressure room, mask on patient when outside room.

Droplet Precautions

- Influenza A or B, Diphtheria, Rubella, Mumps, Pertussis, Scarlet fever, Fifth disease, meningococcal meningitis.
- Mask when within 3 feet of patient, mask on patient when outside room.

Contact Precautions

- RSV, MRSA, VRE, C Difficile, conjunctivitis, E coli, Hepatitis A, shingles, lice, scabies, Chickenpox (Varicella), Hand, foot, and mouth disease, impetigo.
- Gown and gloves when in contact with patient.

16. All the following are treatments for cystic fibrosis (CF) respiratory symptom exacerbation, **EXCEPT**?
    a. Nebulized bronchodilators and hypertonic saline
    b. Magnesium
    c. Chest physiotherapy
    d. Steroids

B – Magnesium is not used in cystic fibrosis. Treatment for cystic fibrosis includes bronchodilators followed by nebulized hypertonic saline to clear airway secretions, steroids for patients with asthma-like symptoms, chest physiotherapy, and possible antibiotics. (ENPC pg. 281)

17. A 2-year-old just arrived in the emergency department in cardiac arrest. The cardiac monitor reveals sinus bradycardia at 30 bpm. High-quality CPR is being performed and intraosseous (IO) access was just obtained. What is your next priority?
    a. Administer epinephrine 0.01 mg/kg IO.
    b. Administer atropine 0.02 mg/kg IO.
    c. Provide transcutaneous pacing.
    d. Apply cricoid pressure.

    A - Epinephrine is the initial medication of choice for PEA. Atropine, transcutaneous pacing, and cricoid pressure are not indicated. (ENPC pg. 112 and PALS pg. 246)

18. On a cold January morning EMS transports a family to the emergency department with complaints of headache, dizziness, shortness of breath, nausea, and vomiting for the past hour. SpO_2 is 100%. You suspect:
    a. Carbon monoxide poisoning
    b. Food poisoning
    c. Viral syndrome
    d. Lead poisoning

    A - Carbon monoxide (CO) is odorless and tasteless and can be emitted from furnaces, automobiles, and portable generators. Pediatric patients get toxic faster due to their increased respiratory rate. Pulse oximetry cannot differentiate oxygenated hemoglobin from carboxyhemoglobin (COHb), so SpO_2 monitoring is unreliable. Treatment is high-flow oxygen until the COHb level drops below 10%. Hyperbaric oxygen therapy may be considered for COHb > 25%. (ENPC pg. 220)

19. For a child that weighs 15 kg, what is the initial defibrillation range?
    a. 7-15 Joules
    b. 15-30 Joules
    c. 30-60 Joules
    d. 50-100 Joules

    C - 30-60 Joules or 2-4 J/kg, up to 10 joules/kg. (ENPC pg. 113 and PALS pg. 92)

20. A fluid bolus for a 15 kg child in severe hypotensive shock from vomiting should be:
    a. 150 mL of an isotonic crystalloid solution over 5-10 minutes
    b. 150 mL of an isotonic crystalloid solution over 10-20 minutes
    c. 300 mL of an isotonic crystalloid solution over 5-10 minutes
    d. 300 mL of an isotonic crystalloid solution over 10-20 minutes

    C - 20 ml/kg (300 mL) over 5 to 10 minutes for severe shock using the "pull-push method" with 20 ml syringes. You may infuse over 20 minutes if not severe shock. Use smaller fluid boluses of 5-10 ml/kg over 10-20 minutes if you suspect cardiogenic shock. Monitor closely for signs of pulmonary edema. (ENPC pg. 108 and PALS pg. 198)

21. Parents bring in a 14-year-old who has been experiencing "fainting spells" during soccer. They saw a neurologist, but all diagnostic tests were negative. The patients older brother died at 16 from a "bad heart". With this history you suspect:
    a. Seizures
    b. Asthma
    c. Long QT syndrome
    d. Acute myocardial infarction

    C - Long QT syndrome (LQTS) is a rare inherited or acquired heart disorder producing fast chaotic heartbeats which may lead to Torsades (TdP) and sudden death. Medications that prolong the QTi include diphenhydramine, haloperidol, erythromycin, quinolones, and ondansetron. Hypokalemia, hypocalcemia, and hypomagnesemia prolong the QTi. (ENPC pg. 106 and PALS pg. 75)

Medications that Prolong QTi

- A AntiArrythmics (Sotalol, Amiodarone)
- B AntiBiotics (Cipro, Levaquin, Erythromycin)
- C AntiCychotics (Haldol, Thorazine, Mellaril)
- D AntiDepressants (Celexa, Lexapro, Effexor)
- E AntiEmetics (Zofran, Droperidol, Reglan)
- F AntiFungals (Ketoconazole)

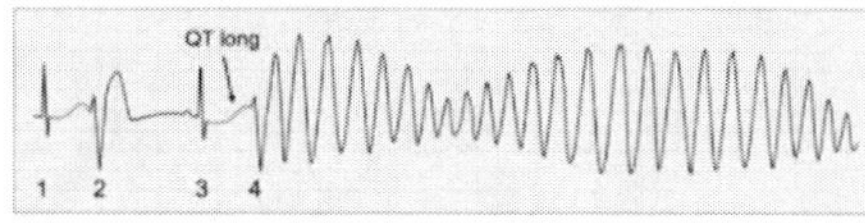

22. A 15-year-old male with a history of Marfan's syndrome arrives in the ED complaining of a sudden onset of shortness of breath. He is in respiratory distress with a respiratory rate of 40, oxygen saturation of 85%, and absent breath sounds on the right side. You suspect:
    a. Dissecting aortic aneurysm
    b. Spontaneous pneumothorax
    c. Congestive heart failure
    d. Huffing of toxic chemicals

    B - Spontaneous pneumothorax. Marfan's is a genetic defect of the connective tissue which is characterized by elongated faces, limbs, fingers, and toes. The risk of spontaneous pneumothorax and aortic aneurysm is higher. These symptoms are suggestive of pneumothorax. (ENPC pg. 282)

23. Coarctation of the aorta and pericardial tamponade are examples of which type of shock?
    a. Obstructive shock
    b. Hypovolemic shock
    c. Cardiogenic shock
    d. Distributive shock

    A – Obstructive shock. Coarctation of the aorta is characterized by narrowing of the aorta at the ductus arteriosus, resulting in increased pressure proximal to the defect (head and upper extremities) and decreased pressure to body and lower extremities. Pericardial tamponade, tension pneumothorax, and massive pulmonary embolism are also examples of obstructive shock. (PALS pgs. 183-186)

24. A 3-year-old patient presents with the following symptoms: fever for the past 7 days, erythematous rash, conjunctivitis, strawberry tongue, and edema of hands and feet. What treatment can the pediatric emergency nurse expect to be ordered?
    a. Tylenol and rest
    b. NSAIDS and antibiotics
    c. Fluids and prostaglandin E1
    d. High-dose aspirin and IV immunoglobulin

    D – The signs and symptoms indicate possible Kawasaki disease, which is treated with **high-dose aspirin and IV immunoglobulin**. Kawasaki disease is a type of pediatric vasculitis with unknown cause, typically in children under the age of five. It can cause many different cardiac complications such as coronary artery aneurysms, stenosis, and cardiomyopathy. (ENPC pg. 152)

25. After a precipitous delivery in the ED the infant is noticed to be cyanotic and tachypneic. The presence of cyanosis in a newly born infant is associated with which congenital defect?
    a. Atrial septal defect
    b. Ventricular septal defect
    c. Patent ductus arteriosus
    d. Transposition of the great vessels

    D - Transposition of the great vessels is characterized by cyanosis and tachycardia at birth since the aorta and pulmonary artery are switched, so oxygenated blood cannot get to the body. Increased risk in advanced maternal age, poor nutrition, or contracting Rubella during pregnancy. (ENPC pg. 89)

26. A 2-day old presents with a heart rate of 200, a RR of 88 breaths/minute and pink, bounding pulses, inspiratory crackles, and a palpable liver. These are signs of what congenital heart defect?
    a. Ventricular Septal Defect (VSD)
    b. Atrial Septal Defect (ASD)
    c. Patent Ductus Arteriosus (PDA)
    d. Tetralogy of Fallot

    C – Patent Ductus Arteriosus (PDA) connects the left pulmonary artery to the aorta to bypass the lungs in utero. Pressure gradients should change with the first few breaths or within 48 hours, but some do not. It results in tachycardia and heart failure. ASD, VSD, and PDA are acyanotic defects. Tetralogy of Fallot and Transposition of the Great Vessels are cyanotic defects. (ENPC pg. 88)

27. The following are signs of ventriculoperitoneal (VP) shunt dysfunction, **EXCEPT**:
    a. Vomiting without nausea
    b. Changes in respiratory rate and pattern
    c. Widening pulse pressure
    d. Left facial drooping.

    D - Facial drooping is a sign of stroke, not shunt dysfunction. The other options are correct as they may be a sign of increased ICP, which may occur with VP shunt dysfunction, particularly obstruction. (ENPC pg. 285)

28. Which of the following is a common sign of meningococcal meningitis in infants?
    a. Petechial rash
    b. Battle's sign
    c. Ipsilateral pupil dilation
    d. Hypertension

    A - Petechial (purple, non-blanching) rash over the body is indicative of meningococcal meningitis, along with restless and inconsolability, opisthotonos, fever, and bulging fontanel. Initiate standard and droplet isolation immediately and prepare for a lumbar puncture in a side-lying position. (ENPC pgs. 151 and 197 and PALS pg. 63)

29. The priority when caring for a patient experiencing a seizure includes:
    a. Maintaining patient safety and administering benzodiazepines.
    b. Intubating the apneic patient and administering Phenytoin (dilantin).
    c. Get labs including a drug screen to determine the cause of the seizure.
    d. Elevating the patient's head 30-45 degrees to decrease intracranial pressure (ICP).

    A – Maintain patient safety and stop seizures. Reduce aspiration risk by turning the patient on side. Stop seizures with IM or IN Midazolam (Versed) if no IV/IO access, or Lorazepam (Ativan) or Midazolam if IV/IO access. Second-line agents include Levetiracetam (Keppra), Fosphenytoin (Cerebryx), Valproic acid (Depakote) Phenytoin, and Phenobarbital. (ENPC pgs. 223-225)

30. A 3-month-old is brought in after having a seizure at home. The family denies head injury or previous history of seizures and the patient is afebrile. Which statement made by the parents may clue the nurse to the cause of the seizure?
    a. "He was recently placed on antibiotics".
    b. "We struggle to afford formula, so we sometimes add extra water to his bottles".
    c. "We recently changed dish detergent".
    d. "He was treated for a PDA when he was a week old".

B – "We sometimes add extra water to his bottles". In infants with an otherwise normal exam, hyponatremia is the leading cause of new onset nonfebrile seizures. Treat with h3% hypertonic saline. (ENPC pg. 90)

31. A 3-day old neonate is brought to the pediatric ED after having a seizure. Shortly after arrival, the patient begins seizing again. The parents reported that the infant has been fussy and has not been latching well to the breast. After protecting the airway, what is the next best action to treat the most likely cause of the seizure?
    a. Draw labs to assess for hyponatremia and administer hypertonic saline IV.
    b. Check blood glucose to assess for hypoglycemia and administer dextrose IV.
    c. Administer isotonic fluid bolus.
    d. Draw blood cultures and administer antibiotics.

B – Check blood glucose as hypoglycemia is the primary metabolic disorder found in neonates. (ENPC pg. 86)

NEOSECRETS Newborn Abnormalities

- **N** iNborn errors of metabolism (hypoglycemia, hyperammonemia)
- **E** Electrolyte abnormalities
- **O** Overdose
- **S** Seizures
- **E** Endocrine (hypoglycemia)
- **C** Cardiac abnormalities (ductal dependent lesions)
- **R** Recipe (incorrect mixing of formula)
- **E** Enteric (malrotation, pyloric stenosis, Hirschsprung)
- **T** Trauma (accidental or non accidental)
- **S** Sepsis

32. What is the most common cause of pediatric acute ischemic stroke?
    a. Congenital atrial fibrillation with patent ductus arteriosus
    b. Von Willebrand's
    c. Sickle Cell Disease
    d. Kawasaki Disease

C – Sickle cell disease leads to stroke in 10% of children with the disease. Sickle cell disease is an inherited blood disorder with abnormal shaped red blood cells that block blood flow. Vaso-occlusive crisis causes excruciating pain. Acute chest syndrome causes shortness of breath and chest pain. The use of hydroxyurea, stem cell transplants, and prophylactic antibiotics have increased outcomes. (ENPC pgs. 282-283)

33. A mother brings in her 1-month-old "with a heart problem" because he "is blue". The infant is cyanotic and crying, but there is no respiratory distress, and lungs are clear. You suspect:
    a. A "Tet Spell"
    b. Congestive heart failure (CHF)
    c. Bronchiolitis
    d. Methemoglobinemia

A - A **"Tet Spell"** from a yet unrepaired Tetralogy of Fallot defect. Tetralogy is the most common cyanotic congenital heart defect. It included a ventricular septal defect, right ventricular outflow tract obstruction, an overriding aorta, and right ventricular hypertrophy. Profound cyanosis occurs from spasms of the muscles around the pulmonary arteries, resulting in a major decrease in pulmonary blood flow. Treatment consists of placing the infant in a knee chest position, oxygen, and morphine. (ENPC pgs. 88-89)

34. A 6-year-old 20-kg female is being evaluated in the emergency department after a syncopal episode. The child is responsive to loud voice, has a respiratory rate of 26 with equal bilateral breath sounds, capillary refill of 3 seconds, pale skin, blood pressure of 76/44, and has a heart rate of 150 bpm in a regular cardiac rhythm with a QRS 0.10 second. What is the treatment priority?
    a. Ask the child to push the plunger out of a 10 mL syringe by blowing on the tip.
    b. Administer Adenosine 2 mg rapid IV bolus followed by a 5-10 mL NS flush.
    c. Consider sedation and perform synchronized cardioversion at 10 to 20 joules.
    d. Administer a 400 mL isotonic crystalloid solution IV over 20 minutes.

C – **Consider sedation and synchronize cardiovert at 0.5 to 1 joule/kg** (10-20 joules) to treat ventricular tachycardia (VT - QRS > 0.09). Vagal maneuvers are utilized in supraventricular tachycardia (SVT), not VT. Adenosine is administered in stable tachycardia, but this child shows signs/symptoms of cardiopulmonary compromise (altered mental status, delayed capillary refill, and hypotension). Fluid resuscitation is used to treat sinus tachycardia, not ventricular tachycardia. (PALS pgs. 249-259)

35. A baseball player takes a direct hit to the chest during the game and immediately collapses. The off-duty pediatric emergency nurse knows the immediate concern is cardiac arrest from ventricular fibrillation or asystole from which disorder?
    a. Prolonged QTi
    b. Wolff-Parkinson-White
    c. Brugada Syndrome
    d. Commotio Cordis

D – **Commotio Cordis** occurs when the precordial area of the chest is struck during the refractory period of the cardiac conduction cycle (T wave) resulting in ventricular fibrillation or asystole. Early bystander CPR, early defibrillation with an AED, and activation of emergency medical services increases the chances of survival. (PALS pg. 75)

36. A 10-month-old child presents to the ED. The patient's mother states that a few hours ago he suddenly became inconsolable and is crying with his knees drawn to his chest. The patient has had two episodes of vomiting with a distended abdomen. Your assessment reveals a distended abdomen with a palpable sausage-shaped mass and "currant jelly" looking stool in the diaper. What test does the nurse anticipate the doctor ordering to confirm this patient's diagnosis?
    a. CT of the abdomen
    b. X-ray of the abdomen
    c. Air or contrast enema
    d. Ultrasound of the abdomen

C – Air or contrast (barium) enema should immediately be performed since the patient is exhibiting symptoms of intussusception. This can both diagnose and treat intussusception, which is described as the telescoping of a segment of bowel into itself. Air or contrast enema is not recommended if signs and symptoms of shock are present. There is risk of bowel perforation and surgical intervention may be required if the enema fails to resolve the condition. (ENPC pg. 167)

37. A 2-week-old infant is brought to the ED. The patient's mother states that the patient appears to have lost weight since birth and has had decreased urine output. She also always seems hungry but has nonbilious projectile vomiting shortly after feeding. Your assessment reveals sunken fontanel, dry mucous membranes, and an olive-shaped mass palpable in the right upper quadrant. What diagnosis does the nurse suspect?
    a. Pyloric Stenosis
    b. Intussusception
    c. Diaphragmatic hernia
    d. Volvulus

    A – Pyloric stenosis often presents in infants 2-6 weeks old with the symptoms described above. Diagnosis can be made via ultrasound and treatment involves a surgical consult for pyloromyotomy. ED management revolves around replenishing fluids and addressing electrolyte imbalances. (ENPC pg. 167)

38. A 3-week-old infant is brought to the emergency department by her parents. The patient's father states that the patient has been fussy with bilious vomiting and blood in her stool. The nurse suspects intestinal volvulus. What treatment plan does she anticipate?
    a. Antibiotics and antiemetics
    b. Air or contrast enema and IV fluids
    c. Gastric decompression and immediate surgical intervention
    d. IV fluids and Protonix infusion

    C – Treatment is **gastric decompression and immediate surgical intervention**. Intestinal volvulus is when loops of bowel twist around each other. Malrotation is a congenital condition in which the intestines have an abnormal rotation which often leads to volvulus and compression of the mesenteric artery, which compromises blood supply to the intestines. Volvulus most often presents within the first month of life but does present as late as age 5. Any time bilious emesis is presented, emergent evaluation for bowel obstruction should occur. (ENPC pg. 169)

39. A 4-month-old infant presents with a history of constipation since birth, abdominal distention, and vomiting. The mother reports foul-smelling, stringy stools. You suspect:
    a. Necrotizing enterocolitis
    b. Intussusception
    c. Hirschsprung's disease
    d. Omphalitis

    C - **Hirschsprung's disease** (aganglionic megacolon) is a congenital disorder of bowel motility because of lack of nerve innervation. It is seen mostly in males, increased risk in children with Down's Syndrome. Necrotizing enterocolitis presents within the first 30 days of life. Omphalitis is an infection of the umbilical stump. (ENPC pgs. 175-176)

40. A 12-year-old patient presents to the ED after rolling over his handlebars on his bike 2 days ago. The patient states that he felt fine after the incident, but now complains of pain to the left shoulder and assessment reveals ecchymosis to the left upper quadrant of the abdomen. What injury do you suspect?
    a. Pancreatic injury
    b. Liver laceration
    c. Spleen laceration
    d. Ruptured bowel

    C – Left shoulder pain (Kehr's sign) and left upper quadrant ecchymosis should raise suspicion for **spleen injury**. The spleen is often injured after blunt trauma such as MVC, sports injuries, and handlebar injuries. Patients sometimes have delayed symptoms due to the spleen being encapsulated. The spleen is a very vascular organ so there is a risk for severe internal bleeding. Most stable patients are treated nonoperatively and observed with serial hemoglobin levels to monitor bleeding. (ENPC pg. 142)

41. A nurse is providing discharge teaching to a 13-year-old patient with celiac disease. Additional discharge teaching is required if the patient makes which statement?
    a. "I should avoid foods containing gluten, such as wheat, barley, and rye".
    b. "If I eat something I should avoid, I might experience diarrhea, constipation, abdominal distention, and pain".
    c. "Not following the appropriate diet can lead to malnutrition as I won't be able to properly absorb nutrients".
    d. "Celiac disease is an allergy to gluten. I should carry an epi-pen in case of emergency".

    D – Celiac disease is a **non-IgE immune-mediated response** in the intestines when exposed to gluten. You do not need to carry an epi pen. (ENPC pg. 167)

42. A 12-year-old patient was trapped under a fallen tree for 4 hours before his parents found him in the woods behind their house. The patient has crush injuries to bilateral lower extremities. Over the next couple of days, this patient is most likely to develop:
    a. Massive hemothorax
    b. Abdominal Compartment syndrome
    c. Tension pneumothorax
    d. Rhabdomyolysis

    D – Rhabdomyolysis is the rapid breakdown of skeletal muscle due to injury to the muscle tissue. The breakdown of muscle results in a release of myoglobin into the bloodstream, which can damage the kidneys, leading to kidney failure. S/S include dark red to brown urine, muscle pain and weakness. Swelling of damaged muscle occasionally leads to compartment syndrome. (TNCC 8th edition pgs. 198 and 227)

43. A 15-year-old patient presents to the emergency department complaining of abdominal pain, and frequent loose stools with bloody diarrhea, What condition does the nurse suspect?
    a. Appendicitis
    b. Inflammatory bowel disease
    c. Pancreatitis
    d. Meckel's diverticulum

    B – Inflammatory bowel disease (IBD) such as Crohn's disease and ulcerative colitis. The peak incidence of IBD occurs in individuals between 15 and 30 years of age. Other symptoms include tenesmus (sensation to pass stool despite an empty bowel) and perianal fistulas. Appendicitis symptoms include periumbilical pain that radiates to the right lower quadrant and rebound tenderness. Children with cystic fibrosis may be predisposed to pancreatitis. Meckel's diverticulum causes painless dark stools. (ENPC pgs. 182-183)

44. Which of the following patients requires immediate surgical intervention?
    a. A patient with an open radial fracture, bleeding controlled via direct pressure by EMS prior to arrival.
    b. A patient complaining of sudden, severe inguinal pain that worsens with elevation of the testicles.
    c. A patient complaining of scrotal pain which is relieved with elevation.
    d. A neonate with projectile, non-bilious vomiting.

    B – Testicular torsion is a surgical emergency to prevent loss of testicular function. Signs and symptoms include sudden onset of severe inguinal pain, nausea and vomiting, pain worse with elevation of the testicle, loss of the cremasteric reflex. The affected testicle may appear red, swollen, and elevated. Doppler reveals reduced or absent blood flow. (ENPC pgs. 184-185)

45. Which of the following are signs and symptoms of epididymitis?
    a. Prolonged penile erection with severe inguinal pain.
    b. Sudden, severe onset of inguinal pain that worsens with elevation.
    c. Gradual onset of scrotal pain that is relieved with elevation, urethral discharge.
    d. Gradual onset of scrotal pain that worsens with elevation, urethral discharge.

    C – Epididymitis is an acute bacterial infection often caused by Chlamydia. It is characterized by s**crotal pain with a gradual onset that is relieved with elevation (Prehn's sign), urinary frequency, and urethral**

discharge. Evaluate for STI's, treat with antibiotics and NSAIDS. Obtain ultrasound if torsion is suspected. (ENPC pg. 191)

46. Primary syphilis is characterized by painless lesions around the external genitalia, anus, or vagina. To prevent long term effects of secondary and tertiary syphilis, treat the sexually transmitted infection with which antibiotic?
    a. Penicillin
    b. Ceftriaxone
    c. Doxycycline
    d. Antiviral therapy

    A – Penicillin is the recommended treatment for syphilis unless the patient is allergic. Ceftriaxone is the first-line treatment for *Neisseria gonorrhea*. Doxycycline or azithromycin is used to treat *Chlamydia trachomatis*. Antiviral therapy is used to treat genital herpes. (ENPC pg. 191)

47. Serology testing is performed to diagnose which sexually transmitted infection?
    a. Human papillomavirus (HPV)
    b. *Neisseria gonorrhea*
    c. *Chlamydia trachomatis*
    d. Syphilis

    D – Syphilis requires serology (blood) testing. (ENPC pg. 186)

48. Which of the following is INCORRECT regarding foreign body ingestion?
    a. Ingested superabsorbent polymers (expandable bath toys) can result in bowel obstruction.
    b. Administer 5 to 10 mL of honey to the symptomatic child who ingested a button battery.
    c. Fishing weights may lead to acute lead poisoning.
    d. Rupture of balloons from "body packing" can cause acute drug toxicity.

    B – Do not administer honey to the symptomatic (vomiting or hematemesis) child, keep them NPO for surgery. Honey can be administered to the asymptomatic child to neutralize the chemical exposure at the site. (ENPC pgs. 177-179)

49. A 7-year-old patient presents to the ED with her parents complaining of bruising and petechiae. The patient has no allergies, takes no medications, and she has no medical problems, except that she is currently recovering from the flu. Labs are drawn and everything appears to be normal except for a platelet level of 75,000. What condition does the nurse suspect?
    a. Hemophilia
    b. Idiopathic Thrombocytopenia Purpura
    c. Henoch-Schoenlein Purpura
    d. Sickle cell anemia

    B – Idiopathic thrombocytopenia purpura (ITP) is a rapid decrease in platelets while other labs are normal, often following a viral illness. It often resolves on its own but can be treated with steroids to decrease immune response that is breaking down platelets, IVIG to rapidly increase platelet count. Platelet transfusions are reserved for life-threatening bleeding. (ENPC pg. 196)

50. Which of the following is described as vasculitis with a purpuric rash and fever due to an autoimmune reaction that primarily affects the small vessels in the joints, skin, and kidneys?
    a. Hemophilia
    b. Idiopathic Thrombocytopenia Purpura
    c. Henoch-Schoenlein Purpura
    d. Sickle cell anemia

    C – Henoch-Schoenlein Purpura (HSP) is most seen in children between 3-10 years old. It is considered idiopathic but is often seen after viral and bacterial infections. Treatment is supportive and usually consists of hydration, rest, and pain management. (ENPC pg. 195)

51. Caregivers report their 6-month-old has been "running a fever, throwing up, and crying a lot". The nurse assesses a tense fontanelle, shrill cry, and petechial rash. The nurse should gather the following information:
    a. Exposure to smoking.
    b. Dilution of formula.
    c. Family history of eczema.
    d. *Hemophilus influenza* type B (HIB) immunization.

D – HIB immunization has decreased the rate of bacterial meningitis and can be given at 6 weeks of age. The nurse should inquire which started first, the fever or the rash, if the child has traveled abroad recently, and if the child has been exposed to anyone actually or potentially ill. Standard and droplet precautions should be initiated. The nurse should prepare for a lumbar puncture. (ENPC pgs. 151-152 and 195-196)

52. A patient with sickle cell anemia presents to the emergency department complaining of pain in extremities and priapism. Vital signs are normal. The provider concludes that the patient is likely experiencing a vaso-occlusive crisis. What orders does the nurse anticipate receiving for this patient?
    a. IV fluids, analgesics, and warm packs for pain control.
    b. IV fluids and cold packs for pain control.
    c. Steroids and oxygen administration.
    d. IV fluids, steroids, analgesics.

A – Treatment for vaso-occlusive crisis includes **IV fluids** to dilute blood and improve perfusion and **pain control**. Use **warm packs**, not cold packs which might make the condition worse, and determine what has worked for the patient's pain in the past. (ENPC pgs. 282-283)

53. Which of the following patients is at increased risk for spinal cord injury with trauma?
    a. A 6-year-old patient with down syndrome.
    b. An 8-year-old patient with sickle cell disease.
    c. A 4-year-old with cystic fibrosis.
    d. A 2-year-old with an allergy to peanuts.

A – Patients with **down syndrome** often have atlantoaxial instability which increases their risk of spinal cord injury. (ENPC pg. 282)

54. A child initially diagnosed with SARS-CoV-2 has progressed to multisystem inflammatory disease. What medical treatment is indicated for the critically ill child refractory to epinephrine and dopamine?
    a. High-dose aspirin.
    b. Insertion of a ventricular assist device.
    c. Extracorporeal membrane oxygenation (ECMO).
    d. Insertion of a ventriculoatrial shunt.

C – ECMO may be used for critically ill patients who are not responding to IVIG, steroids, epinephrine or norepinephrine, and dopamine or dobutamine. Overall mortality is low at 1% to 2%. (ENPC pgs. 154-155)

55. A mother runs into the emergency department with her 6-year-old child who is unresponsive. The child has a history of type 1 diabetes and has a "stomach bug" for the past 3 days. Blood glucose reading is 32mg/dL. The following medication choices are appropriate for this patient, **EXCEPT:**
    a. Glucagon 0.5 to 1 mg intramuscularly if IV access is not available.
    b. 5 mL/kg of D 50%.
    c. 2.5 to 5 mL/kg of $D_{10}W$.
    d. 1 to 2 mL/kg of $D_{25}W$.

B – D 50% is too concentrated for a pediatric patient. Hypoglycemia is defined as a blood glucose reading below 70 mg/dL in a pediatric patient. For conscious and alert patients, 10-20 grams of oral carbohydrates are appropriate. For unconscious patients, dextrose IV. IM glucagon can be administered if there is no IV access available. Reevaluate the blood sugar 15 minutes after treatment and hourly until it is stabilized. (ENPC pg. 211)

56. What type of intracranial hemorrhage typically results in irritability, vomiting, a slow, steady decline in level of consciousness, and new onset seizures?
    a. Intracerebral
    b. Epidural
    c. Subdural
    d. Subarachnoid

C – A **subdural hemorrhage** is venous bleeding between the dura mater and arachnoid membranes. It may be the result of shaken baby syndrome and abuse. Subarachnoid hemorrhage can also occur in neonates at this time of birth. (ENPC pg. 259)

57. A 13-year-old patient suffers from a concussion. During discharge teaching, the patient asks when he can play football again. What is the appropriate response from the nurse?
    a. He can begin playing again once he is symptom-free for 24 hours.
    b. He should follow a graduated return-to-play protocol.
    c. He will not be able to play full contact sports for at least 6 weeks.
    d. He will not be able to play until he has a clear CT scan.

B – It is recommended that patients **follow the graduated return-to-play** protocol after suffering from a concussion. Activity is gradually increased as the patient can reach each step without symptoms. Additional discharge education includes acetaminophen only for pain, and cognitive brain rest until the symptoms resolve. (ENPC pg.140)

58. A 3-month-old born at 35 weeks gestation just started daycare. Assessment findings include a runny nose, cough, and retractions. Wheezing and crackles are audible throughout. Pulse oximetry shows a saturation of 90% oxygen. Which of the following is the priority intervention?
    a. Racemic epinephrine
    b. Corticosteroids
    c. Antibiotic therapy
    d. Oxygen via high-flow nasal cannula (HFNC)

D – **Oxygen via high-flow nasal cannula** or non-invasive positive pressure ventilation may prevent progression from respiratory distress from **bronchiolitis** to respiratory failure. The risk of bronchiolitis increases with exposure to smoke, crowded households, siblings in the home, and daycare attendance. Bronchiolitis is most often caused by the respiratory syncytial virus (RSV). Treatment includes antipyretics and oxygen, not bronchodilators, epinephrine, corticosteroids, or nebulized hypertonic saline. (ENPC pgs. 119-120)

59. A 15-month-old child is carried into the emergency department by her caregivers who report she choked while playing. Coughing and stridor are assessed. Which is the priority intervention?
    a. Nebulized racemic epinephrine.
    b. Five back blows, then 5 chest thrusts
    c. Bronchoscopy
    d. Abdominal thrusts

C – **Bronchoscopy** is needed to facilitate removal of the foreign body. BLS is not required currently since the child is coughing. (ENPC pgs. 119-120)

60. The Monro-Kellie hypothesis states the skull is a finite space that houses the brain, blood, and cerebral spinal fluid (CSF). If one component increases, pressure is applied to the brain. Which of the following is a late sign of hydrocephalus in infants?
    a. Higher-pitched cry
    b. Seizures
    c. Widening cranial sutures
    d. Sunset eyes

B – **Seizures** are a late sign of hydrocephalus. Children with hydrocephalus are often treated with a ventriculoperitoneal (VP) shunt. (ENPC pgs. 231-233)

61. A 5-year-old child is brought to the ED by her parents with abdominal pain and vomiting. Assessment reveals parched lips, tachycardia, and a fruity odor to her breath. The nurse suspects which endocrine disorder?
    a. Hypoglycemia
    b. Diabetes insipidus (DI)
    c. Diabetic ketoacidosis (DKA)
    d. Hyperosmolar hyperglycemic state (HHS)

C – Thirty percent of DKA is diagnosed in the ED, due to increased thirst, fruity breath, and increased respiration. Children ages 4-7 are diagnosed often. Blood glucose is typically > 200 mg/dl, pH < 7.3, with ketones in urine. Treatment focuses on correcting hypovolemia, and infusing insulin until the anion gap closes. (ENPC pgs. 224-226)

62. A child falls from a tree and briefly loses consciousness. He arrives in the emergency department awake and alert, but loses consciousness again while in CT. You suspect which type of intracranial hemorrhage?
    a. Epidural
    b. Subdural
    c. Subarachnoid
    d. Intracerebral

A - Epidural hemorrhage is arterial (middle meningeal artery) bleeding between the skull and the dura, so bleeding rapidly progresses. S/S: include headache, nausea, vomiting, with a possible lucid period. (TNCC 8th edition pg. 107)

63. The following medications can be administered to decrease cerebral edema after traumatic brain injury, **EXCEPT**:
    a. Mannitol
    b. Dexamethasone
    c. Furosemide
    d. Hypertonic saline

B – Dexamethasone is incorrect. Osmotic (Mannitol) and loop (furosemide) diuretics may be administered to decrease cerebral edema. Hypertonic saline may be considered if they fail. Corticosteroids are not used in the treatment of TBI. (ENPC pg. 139)

64. A 5-year-old patient involved in an MVC complains of numbness of bilateral lower extremities. A CT scan is obtained, and no vertebral injury is seen. The patient is still unable to feel his lower extremities. What test is indicated next?
    a. X-ray of the cervical spine
    b. MRI of the spine
    c. NEXUS
    d. None, the patient is experiencing spinal shock which will resolve on its own.

B – MRI of the spine. SCIWORA (spinal cord injury without radiographic abnormality) may occur in pediatric patients due to hyperextension injuries. Pediatric patients have more flexible vertebral ligaments that may allow the spinal cord to become injured without fracturing vertebrae. MRI can be used to determine the extent of the injury not able to be seen on x-ray or CT. NEXUS criteria are used to determine whether a potential spinal injury can be ruled out clinically without diagnostic imaging. (TNCC 8th edition pg. 235)

65. You are assessing a 14-year-old patient that EMS brought to the ED after a MVC in which the patient was ejected from the vehicle. The patient is warm and flushed and states that he cannot move his arms or legs. The right forearm was splinted by EMS, and they reported obvious deformity. Vital signs are as follows: B/P 79/42, HR 45, RR 18, SpO2 95% on room air. What kind of shock is this patient most likely experiencing?
    a. Hypovolemic
    b. Distributive
    c. Cardiogenic
    d. Obstructive

B – Neurogenic shock is a form of **distributive shock**. Although trauma patients are at risk of hypovolemic shock due to bleeding, this patient does not show evidence of extensive blood loss. The decreased heart rate with likely spinal cord injury is the hallmark sign of neurogenic shock. (ENPC pg. 103)

66. A 5-year-old is brought to the ED after being struck in the eye during a baseball game. Your assessment reveals periorbital edema, hyperesthesia of the cheek and upper lip, diplopia, and limited upward gaze. What injury do you suspect?
    a. Hyphema
    b. Globe rupture
    c. Retinal detachment
    d. Orbital fracture

D – An **orbital fracture** will present with periorbital edema, hyperesthesia (increased sensation) of the cheek and upper lip, diplopia, enophthalmos (inward eye displacement), and limited upward gaze due to entrapment of the inferior rectus. Early ophthalmic assessment is important to rule out damage to the globe and retina. Immediate surgical intervention is warranted for fractures causing diplopia, nerve entrapment or severe enophthalmos. (TNCC 8th edition pgs. 112-113)

67. Which chemical substance is most likely to cause a more severe injury to the eye?
    a. Bleach
    b. Sulfuric acid
    c. Vinegar
    d. Citric acid

A – **Bleach** is a strong alkali and alkali injuries are more severe than acid injuries. Immediate irrigation is indicated for both acid and alkali injuries. Immediate, thorough irrigation with copious amounts of normal saline or lactated ringers is indicated and should be continued until pH of the eye is normal at 7.4. LR may be more comfortable for the patient as the pH is closer to human tears. Avoid patching the eye due to risk of infection. (TNCC 8th edition pg.114)

68. A 16-year-old patient presents to the ED after being punched in the eye during a fight. The patient complains of right eye pain with vision loss and nausea. Your assessment reveals blood in the anterior chamber of the eye. What injury do you suspect?
    a. Globe rupture
    b. Orbital fracture
    c. Hyphema
    d. Retinal detachment

C – A **hyphema** is a collection of blood in the anterior chamber of the eye. An "eight ball hyphema" is the total filling of the chamber with blood. Treatment included bed rest with the head of the bed elevated to 30-45 degrees. Rebleeding may occur, and usually occurs within 3 to 5 days after initial injury. Instruct patient to return to the ED if signs of rebleeding occur. (ENPC pg.79)

69. A 7-year-old patient presents via EMS with a stick penetrating the left eye after tripping in the woods while playing. What is the most appropriate action for the management for the penetrating object?
    a. Remove the object carefully, while instructing the patient to hold the eye still.
    b. Place tetracaine drops in the eye to decrease pain.
    c. Use a cup to stabilize the object.
    d. Use gauze to apply pressure while stabilizing the object.

C – Use a **cup to stabilize the object** while avoiding putting pressure on the globe. Avoid moving the object. Cover the unaffected eye to prevent movement of the affected eye. Avoid the use of eye drops. (TNCC 8th edition pg. 113)

70. A 17-year-old patient presents to the ED after being involved in an MVC. The patient complains of eye pain and loss of vision to his right eye after his face struck the steering wheel. Your assessment reveals a small laceration of the eyelid and a teardrop-shaped pupil. What injury do you suspect?
    a. Globe rupture
    b. Orbital fracture
    c. Hyphema
    d. Retinal detachment

A – **Globe rupture** may be due to penetrating or blunt trauma to the face due to the sudden increase in intraocular pressure. Typical presentation reveals a teardrop shaped or irregular pupil. Appropriate interventions include placing a rigid protective eye shield. Medicate the patient to prevent anything that increases intraocular pressure such as vomiting, pain, and agitation. Avoid putting eye drops in the eye. Surgical intervention is required. (TNCC 8th edition pg. 113)

71. What type of spinal fracture is often associated with lap belt injuries?
    a. Chance Fracture
    b. Clavicle fracture
    c. Hangman's fracture
    d. Atlas fracture

A – A **chance fracture** results from excessive flexion of the spine, often associated with lap belt injuries and seen in **T12-L2**. Hangman's fracture is a fracture of C2. C1 is also known as the Atlas. The clavicle is not part of the spine. (ENPC pg. 131)

72. A 11-year-old female patient is brought to the ED via EMS after falling from a ladder. The patient is awake and oriented x2, respirations even and unlabored with no obvious external bleeding. Vital signs are 85/44, heart rate 130, RR 20, SpO_2 99% on room air. During your secondary survey, you note an unstable pelvis with blood oozing from the meatus. All other assessments appear to be normal. The following are appropriate interventions for this patient, **EXCEPT**:
    a. Administer crystalloid bolus at 20mL/kg and be prepared to initiate blood transfusion.
    b. Apply a pelvic binder to stabilize the pelvis.
    c. Insert a urinary catheter for accurate measurement of urine output to ensure proper resuscitation.
    d. Maintain cervical spine precautions until CT rules out cervical spine injury.

C – Bleeding from the urethra indicates possible urethra or bladder injury, which are common with unstable pelvic fractures. **Avoid placing an indwelling catheter if a bladder or urethral injury may be present.** (ENPC pg. 135)

73. A patient presents with an injury to his left leg. In the x-ray report, the radiologist describes the fracture present as Salter-Harris Type V. The pediatric emergency nurse knows that this indicates:
    a. There is a fracture straight across the growth plate, this is the least severe type and should not interfere with future growth.
    b. There is a fracture below the growth plate, it is somewhat severe and may interfere with future growth.
    c. There is a fracture through the growth plate, it is severe and will likely affect future growth.
    d. The fracture has crushed the growth plate, this has the worst prognosis and future growth will be stunted.

D – Fractures are classified from Salter-Harris I to V with **V being the most severe, crushing the growth plate**, with the worst prognosis and future growth will be stunted. (ENPC pg. 143)

74. A 10-year-old patient returns to the ED after having had a splint placed for a forearm fracture. The patient is complaining of increased, unrelenting pain to the injury site, worse with passive movement. The patient has a distal pulse. Which of the following best describes the appropriate plan of action for the nurse?
    a. Assure the patient that everything is OK because there is still a pulse present, that pain is a normal finding, and request that the doctor order a stronger pain medication.
    b. Remove the splint, place the extremity at a neutral position level with the heart, and prepare for an emergent fasciotomy.
    c. Remove the splint, elevate the extremity to decrease pressure, and prepare for an emergent fasciotomy.
    d. Remove the splint and elevate the extremity to relieve external pressure which is causing the patient's pain.

B – Remove the splint since you suspect compartment syndrome. The primary symptom is **pain out of proportion** to the injury with passive movement. Place the extremity **at the level of the heart (neutral position)**; avoid elevating the extremity because it decreases arterial blood flow and worsens venous congestion. The absence of distal pulses is a late sign which confirms compromised circulation. A fasciotomy may be necessary to relieve the pressure and allow blood flow until swelling subsides. (TNCC 8th edition pgs. 196-198)

75. You are caring for a 6-year-old burn patient who weighs 20 kg with a 30% BSA partial thickness thermal burn. According to the American Burn Association, how much fluid should this pediatric patient receive in the first 8 hours?
    a. 900 mL
    b. 1,2000 mL
    c. 1,800 mL
    d. 2,400 mL

A – 900 mL. The American Burn Association recommends **3 mL x weight in kg x % TBSA** = total fluids over 24 hours for thermal burns. Half of the total fluids are to be administered in the first 8 hours from the time of the burn and the second half over the remaining 16 hours. 3mL x 20 x 30% = 1,800; 1,800 / 2 = 900. Ensure that the fluids are warmed to maintain normothermia. (ENPC pg. 137)

76. You are treating a patient who has been burned with hydrofluoric acid. After thoroughly irrigating the burn, what medication should be applied to the burn?
    a. 2.5% calcium gluconate gel.
    b. 1% silver sulfadiazine cream.
    c. Bacitracin ointment.
    d. No medication should be applied, wrap the burn in dry sterile dressings.

A – When treating hydrofluoric acid burns, **2.5% calcium gluconate gel** should be applied to the burn after irrigating for 30 minutes or until pain relief. (TNCC 8th edition pg. 228)

Special Considerations (25 Exam Questions, 25 Samples)

1. You are resuscitating a neonate on arrival. Positive pressure ventilation is being performed via an endotracheal tube, and chest compressions have been initiated for a heart rate below 60. After one minute of chest compressions, the heart rate still has not increased. What is your next step?
    a. Stimulate the infant.
    b. Initiate dopamine infusion.
    c. Administer epinephrine.
    d. Administer fluid bolus.

    C – Epinephrine is the first medication in NRP to be administered after 60 seconds of chest compressions with no increase in heart rate. (NRP)

2. At what rate should breaths be administered during the initial stages of neonatal resuscitation?
    a. 35-45
    b. 40-60
    c. 50-60
    d. 60-80

    B – Positive pressure breaths should be given at a rate of **40-60 breaths per minute**. (ENPC pg. 85)

3. A neonate has just been delivered. He is flaccid, and not breathing or crying. What are the next steps that should be taken?
    a. Warm and dry the patient, position the airway, and stimulate.
    b. Warm and dry the patient, stimulate, initiate positive pressure ventilation.
    c. Stimulate the patient, initiate positive pressure ventilation, begin chest compressions.
    d. Initiate positive pressure ventilation, check for a pulse, and begin chest compressions.

    A – The initial steps of neonatal resuscitation for a non-vigorous newborn are to **warm and dry the neonate, position the airway, clear secretions if needed, and stimulate**. (ENPC pg. 84)

4. You are providing positive pressure ventilation to a bradycardic neonate just after birth. What is the best indicator of successful positive-pressure ventilation (PPV)?
    a. Patient's skin is turning pink.
    b. Increasing heart rate.
    c. SpO_2 of 100% five minutes after birth.
    d. The neonate is becoming more alert.

    B – Increasing heart rate is the best indicator of effective positive pressure ventilation in the bradycardic neonate. Target preductal SpO_2 at 5 minutes after birth is 80-85%. (ENPC pg. 85)

5. Which statement made by the new parent requires further education?
    a. I feed her formula because of the medications I am taking.
    b. She has reflux so I always put her to sleep on her stomach to prevent aspiration if she vomits.
    c. Her car seat is secured in the back seat and is rear facing.
    d. I keep her crib clear of pillows and blankets to prevent suffocation.

    B – Infants should always be placed on their **"back to sleep"**, until they are old enough to roll over on their own. The crib should be kept clear of loose blankets and pillows and bed-sharing should be avoided. Children should be placed in rear-facing car seats until they are at least 2-3 years old.

6. A 2-year-old patient is brought to your ED after being found unresponsive in a pool. CPR is in progress. The pediatric emergency nurse knows that the family should be:
   a. Placed in a private waiting room and updated frequently.
   b. Monitored by security to prevent a dangerous situation due to emotional outbursts.
   c. Allowed to stay at the bedside with a staff member whose role is to communicate with the family.
   d. Kept in the hallway with the door closed so they do not see anything traumatic.

   C – The **family should be allowed to remain at bedside if they wish**. A staff member should be dedicated to communicating with them and answering questions. Patient- and family-centered care is based on the concepts of information sharing, respect and honoring differences, partnership and collaboration, negotiation, and care specific to the patient and the family. (ENPC pg.75)

7. Which of the following is appropriate when caring for a patient with Autism?
   a. Frequently change providers as the patient will lose trust after painful procedures.
   b. Provide a space with a lot of distractions to keep the patient distracted during painful portions of the exam.
   c. Explain procedures in detail prior to performing them.
   d. Place the patient in a room that is protected from sound away from main hallways.

   D – Patients with Autism can become over-stimulated, so a **quiet environment is best**. Maintain consistent team members. Offer noise-canceling headphones, sunglasses, and a weighted blanket. (ENPC pg. 246)

8. A patient with autism spectrum disorder (ASD) was brought in by his mother to be seen for a laceration to his eyelid. The mother states that the patient has been experiencing increased agitation and self-harm over the past few days. All the following are appropriate interventions for this patient, **EXCEPT**:
   a. Place the patient in a low stimulus area.
   b. Avoid touching the patient as much as possible.
   c. Ensure that the patient does not have access to equipment that he could use to hurt himself or others and ensure that the patient is closely monitored.
   d. Have the mother sit in the waiting room and keep security at bedside to prevent the patient from injuring her during an outburst.

   D – Allow the **patient's caregivers to assist with a patient** with ASD, unless the patient is acting violently toward them. Caregivers can provide useful information about the best techniques to gain cooperation and having a trusted caregiver around can help to calm these patients. (ENPC pg. 246)

9. An unresponsive 5-month-old patient is brought to the emergency department after reportedly rolling off a bed. Which assessment finding would cause the nurse to suspect nonaccidental trauma to this patient?
   a. A bruise to the forehead where the patient reportedly hit his head.
   b. A laceration to the forehead with bleeding controlled.
   c. A fractured wrist.
   d. Retinal hemorrhage upon ophthalmic assessment.

   D –Retinal hemorrhages, posterior rib fractures, and subdural hemorrhages are the most common findings in shaken impact syndrome or **abusive head trauma**. (ENPC pg. 257)

10. A 9-year-old who was sexually assaulted 2 months earlier is brought to the ED for outbursts of anger, sleep disturbances, and flashbacks of the abuse. The nurse expects the patient to receive treatment for:
    a. Acute stress reaction
    b. Bipolar disorder
    c. Acute psychosis
    d. Post-traumatic stress disorder (PTSD)

    D – **Post-traumatic stress disorder (PTSD)** begins around 2 months after the event. Other signs of PTSD are hyper alertness and regressive behavior. Place the patient in a low stimulus area. (ENPC pg. 248)

11. A 16-year-old patient presents to the ED. Her mother states she has been experiencing tremors with strange muscle contractions and repetitive movements, slurred speech, and restlessness (akathisia). The patient has a history of schizophrenia and asthma and is currently being treated for strep throat. The mother provides a list of her medications, and the nurse suspects that the symptoms may be related to which of the following:
    a. Haloperidol
    b. Albuterol
    c. Ipratropium
    d. Amoxicillin

    A – The symptoms described are extrapyramidal symptoms (EPS) which are often caused by antipsychotic medications like **haloperidol (Haldol)**. Dystonia (muscle spasms) can be treated with diphenhydramine. Akathisia symptoms may be treated with beta blockers and benzodiazepines. (ENPC pg. 246)

12. A 16-year-old patient presents to the ED via EMS with nausea, vomiting, and diaphoresis. Her parents reported they found an empty bottle of acetaminophen in the patient's room when they tried to get her up for school. The patient states "I just wanted to sleep." What is the appropriate antidote to administer to this patient?
    a. Flumazenil (Romazicon)
    b. N-Acetylcysteine (Acetadote)
    c. Naloxone (Narcan)
    d. Fomepizole (Antizol)

    B – N-Acetylcysteine (Acetadote) is the antidote for acetaminophen overdose. Activated charcoal can be administered within 1 hour of ingestion if the patient is alert. Acetaminophen overdose can lead to severe hepatotoxicity. (ENPC pg. 213)

13. A 14-year-old patient presents to the ED after having a seizure. The patient's mother states that she does not have a history of seizures. The patient is postictal and vital signs are as follows: temp 102.1, HR 155, BP 192/98, RR 8, SpO_2 94%. EKG reveals a prolonged QT interval. Which medication might the patient have overdosed on?
    a. Digoxin
    b. Amitriptyline
    c. Acetaminophen
    d. Hydrocodone

    B – Amitriptyline (Elavil) is a tricyclic antidepressant. TCA's have a narrow margin of safety and toxicity can lead to anticholinergic toxidrome (mydriasis, urinary retention, dry mouth, hyperthermia, hypertension, tachycardia, muscle twitching), QRS prolongation, ventricular dysrhythmias, and seizures. Severe cases can lead to rhabdomyolysis and renal failure. (ENPC pg. 217)

14. A patient presents with Amitriptyline (Elavil) toxicity. All the following medications are appropriate to treat the symptoms, **EXCEPT**:
    a. Sodium bicarbonate
    b. Benzodiazepines
    c. Potassium
    d. Magnesium

    C – Potassium is the incorrect answer. Medications administered for TCA antidepressant toxicity include sodium bicarbonate, lidocaine, magnesium, and benzodiazepines. (ENPC pg. 217)

15. A 17-year-old patient presents to the ED lethargic but arousable after a reported benzodiazepine overdose. The patient is prescribed Ativan that she takes daily for anxiety and states "I just wanted it all to end." The physician orders flumazenil for reversal of the overdose. What is the appropriate response by the nurse?
    a. "I will draw up the flumazenil and administer it intravenously".
    b. "Did you mean to order Narcan instead?"
    c. "I will be sure to administer it intramuscularly".
    d. "This patient takes benzodiazepines daily and may be at risk for seizures. Are you sure that I should give flumazenil?"

D – Clarify the order. Flumazenil is the reversal agent for benzodiazepines, but it is no longer recommended in benzodiazepine dependent patients because it may cause **seizures.** Supportive care of airway, breathing, and circulation and monitoring are usually recommended for treatment of benzodiazepine overdose. (ENPC pg. 213)

16. A pediatric patient who ate a bottle of vitamins with iron was administered deferoxamine, which is a chelating agent. The patient's mother is concerned when the patient's urine appears to be pink in color a few hours later. What is the most appropriate response by the nurse?
    a. "I will let the doctor know. GI bleeding is common with iron overdose".
    b. "That is a common side effect of deferoxamine, and it is harmless".
    c. "We will continue to monitor the patient to see if it gets worse".
    d. "I will talk to the doctor because coagulopathies are an adverse effect that can occur with deferoxamine administration".

B – Deferoxamine is a chelating agent that is the reversal agent for iron. It often turns **urine pink** as it is excreted. (ENPC pgs. 213, 217-218)

17. A 3-year-old patient is brought into the emergency department. The patient's father states that the patient got into the fertilizer while they were outside gardening. The patient presents lethargic with excessive salivation, watery sputum, is incontinent of urine and feces, and vomited prior to arrival. What is the appropriate antidote for this patient?
    a. Flumazenil (Romazicon)
    b. Naloxone (Narcan)
    c. Atropine and Pralidoxime
    d. N-Acetylcysteine (Acetadote)

C –High doses of atropine and Pralidoxime are administered for organophosphate poisoning. Signs and symptoms of organophosphate poisoning are remembered using SLUDGE/BBB (salivation, lacrimation, urination, defecation, GI, emesis, bronchorrhea, bronchospasm, bradycardia) mnemonic. Intubation may be necessary due to airway secretions. (ENPC pg. 222)

18. A 14-year-old patient presents with signs and symptoms of euphoria, mydriasis, tachycardia, hypertension, and hyperthermia after trying cocaine at a friend's house. Which of the following medications is **NOT** appropriate in the management of this patient's symptoms?
    a. Beta blockers
    b. Benzodiazepines
    c. Sodium bicarbonate
    d. Phentolamine

A – Beta blockers are not indicated in the management of cocaine toxicity due to the hypertension that can result from unopposed alpha-adrenergic stimulation. Patients experiencing sympathomimetic toxicity should be monitored for the development of serious conditions such as rhabdomyolysis, stroke, and myocardial infarction. (ENPC pg. 220)

19. Which of the following medications is indicated in the treatment of beta-blocker toxicity?
    a. Flumazenil (Romazicon)
    b. Naloxone (Narcan)
    c. Fomepizole (Antizol)
    d. Glucagon

D – **Glucagon** and calcium are first line antidotes, along with high-dose insulin/glucose/potassium, lipid emulsion, and vasopressors. Glucagon may cause vomiting, so have suction at the bedside. (ENPC pgs. 213 and 217)

20. An 8-year-old presents to the ED with complaints of fever, cough, runny nose, conjunctivitis, and a rash. The patient's mother states that he is unvaccinated. Your assessment reveals a maculopapular rash to the face and shoulders, Koplik spots on the mucous membranes, and a fever of 103. What diagnosis do you suspect?
    a. Mumps
    b. Measles
    c. Diphtheria
    d. Chicken Pox

B – Signs and symptoms of **measles** include "The 3 C's" which are cough, coryza (runny nose), and conjunctivitis. This is accompanied by an erythematous maculopapular rash which starts at the hairline and advances downward toward the face and neck, then to the hands and feet. Koplik spots are small blue-white spots visible on the oral mucosa 1-2 days after the body rash appears. (ENPC pg. 200)

21. Which of the following is characterized by myalgias, parotitis, and orchitis in male patients?
    a. Mumps
    b. Measles
    c. Diphtheria
    d. Chicken pox

A – Mumps. Other symptoms include anorexia, headache, malaise, and low-grade fever. Treatment is mostly supportive. Complications include orchitis and pancreatitis.

22. Which of the following injuries is most suspicious for physical abuse in a 2-year-old child?
    a. A spiral ulnar fracture after reportedly falling off the bed.
    b. Bruises to the arms and legs in various stages of healing.
    c. A hematoma on the forehead after reportedly falling out of a stroller.
    d. Partial thickness burns to the palms after reportedly touching the inside of the oven while his mother was cooking.

A – Spiral fractures are generally caused by twisting injuries, and the injury pattern above is inconsistent with the history. The other injury patterns are appropriate for the patient's age and mechanism of injury. Non-accidental trauma should also be considered when there is a delay in seeking medical care for what appears to be a serious injury, multiple injuries at various stages of healing, bruises to the abdomen and chest (bruises on arms and legs of a 2-year-old is not an unexpected finding for the patient's age), bite marks, **burns with lines of demarcation**, cigarette burns, subdural hematomas or retinal hemorrhages, rib fractures, especially at different chronological stages. (ENPC pg. 257)

23. Congenital Adrenal Hyperplasia (CAH) results in which electrolyte imbalance?
    a. Hypernatremia
    b. Hyperkalemia
    c. Hyperglycemia
    d. Increased serum osmolality

B – **Hyperkalemia**, hyponatremia, and hypoglycemia are seen in CAH due to cortisol deficiency. Infants may exhibit vomiting and signs of shock. Treat with NS, hydrocortisone, and calcium and insulin for hyperkalemia. (ENPC pg. 86)

24. What is the initial sign/symptom of Rickettsia?
    a. Erythema migrans
    b. Nonpruritic macular rash
    c. Severe muscle cramping
    d. Ulcerative rash

B – The initial S/S **Rickettsia (Rocky Mountain Spotted fever) is a nonpruritic macular (flat) rash**. The highest number of cases occur from tick bites in North Carolina and Tennessee. Erythema migrans is common in Lyme's disease. Muscle cramping is common in scorpion stings and black widow spider bites. An ulcerative rash is seen in brown recluse spider bites.

25. What illness begins with an unsteady gait, progressing to symmetrical ascending flaccid paralysis?
    a. Lyme disease
    b. Muscular dystrophy
    c. Tick paralysis
    d. Alpha-gal syndrome

C – The initial symptom of **tick paralysis** is an unsteady gate, progressing to symmetrical ascending flaccid paralysis. The tick toxin is like botulinum toxin and may cause death from respiratory arrest. Lyme disease causes flu-like symptoms and erythema migrans. Progressive muscle weakness is seen in muscular dystrophy (not ascending). Alpha-gal syndrome causes a red meat allergy after a Lone Star tick bite.

TEN 4 FACES P Suspicious Bruises in Children

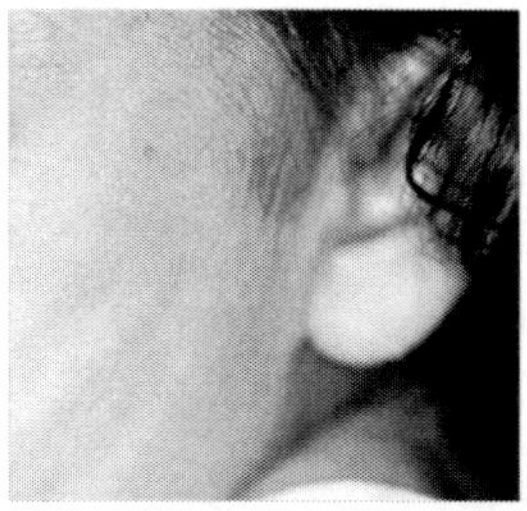

- Torso, Ear, or Neck in children under 4 years of age.
- Frenulum, Auricular, Cheeks, Eyelid, Sclera in infants under 4 months of age.
- Patterned injuries.

Emergency Antidote Chart

Toxin	Antidote
Acetaminophen	N-acetylcysteine (Acetadote)
Tricyclics (TCAs)	Sodium Bicarbonate, Lidocaine
Opioids	Narcan (Naloxone)
Benzodiazepines	Romazicon (Flumazenil) questionable
Ca Channel blockers	Calcium, Glucagon, Insulin
Beta blockers	Glucagon, Insulin
Organophosphates	Atropine/2-PAM
Ethylene glycol	Ethanol or Fomepizole (Antizol)
Iron	Deferoxamine
Sulfonylureas	Dextrose, Octreotide

Multi-System Considerations (12 Exam Questions, 12 Samples)

1. The ideal oxygen saturation after return of spontaneous circulation (ROSC) is:
    a. 90-92%
    b. 90-94%
    c. 94-99%
    d. 98-100%

    C – 94-99%. Titrate oxygen administration to achieve normoxemia, avoiding hypoxemia and hyperoxia. (PALS pg. 263)

2. Which of the following assessment findings may be an indicator of warm septic shock that would **NOT** be found in other forms of shock?
    a. Temperature < 36° C
    b. Capillary refill < 1 second
    c. Hypotension despite fluid resuscitation
    d. Urticaria

    B – Flash (less than 1 second) capillary refill can be an indicator for warm septic shock. Other signs/symptoms include bounding pulses, flushed/hot skin, normal/elevated blood pressure. A temperature of less than 36° C may indicate "cold" septic shock. Hypotension can present in any form of shock; urticaria may be present in anaphylactic shock. (PALS pg. 177)

3. Which of the following is **NOT** a common risk factor for near-drowning (submersion injury)?
    a. Obesity
    b. Lack of supervision
    c. Poor swimming skills
    d. Alcohol or drug abuse

    A – Obesity is NOT a risk factor for near-drowning. Lack of supervision, inability to or poor swimming skills, alcohol or drug abuse, and history of seizures are risk factors for submersion injury. Outcomes are related to length of time submerged.

4. Septic shock is which type of shock?
    a. Hypovolemic shock
    b. Obstructive shock
    c. Cardiogenic shock
    d. Distributive shock

    D – Septic shock is distributive shock. Distributive shock is characterized by a maldistribution of blood volume and blood flow. (PALS pg. 175)

5. Which is correct regarding the pathophysiology of septic shock?
    a. Systemic vascular resistance (SVR) is high.
    b. Preload is high.
    c. Cardiac output is high in early sepsis.
    d. There is a loss of sympathetic tone.

    C – Cardiac output is high in early sepsis or the "warm phase". Distributive shock is characterized by a low systemic vascular resistance (SVR) or afterload. The preload or volume is low due to maldistribution of blood flow and capillary permeability. Neurogenic shock is characterized by a loss of sympathetic tone. (PALS pgs. 175-179)

6. Nausea/vomiting and urticaria in anaphylaxis is due to which physiologic process?
   a. Histamine and mediator release.
   b. Fluid leakage from blood vessels.
   c. Vasodilation from maldistribution of blood flow.
   d. Inadequate blood flowing to the tissues.

   A – Nausea/vomiting and urticaria in anaphylaxis is due to histamine and mediator release. Swelling of tongue is due to fluid leak from blood vessels. Stridor is caused by the inflammatory response. Tachycardia is due to inadequate blood flow to the tissues. Hypotension is due to vasodilation. (PALS pg. 179)

7. Utilizing the 4-2-1 method, what is the hourly maintenance fluid for an 8-kg infant?
   a. 16 mL/hour
   b. 32 mL/hour
   c. 36 mL/hour
   d. 42 mL/hour

   B – Maintenance fluid administration for infants < 10 kg is 4 mL/kg, so 32 mL/hour. (PALS pg. 274)

8. Utilizing the 4-2-1 method, what is the hourly maintenance fluid for a 15-kg child?
   a. 30 mL/hour
   b. 40 mL/hour
   c. 50 mL/hour
   d. 60 mL/hour

   C – Maintenance fluid administration for children 10-20 kg is 40 mL/hour + 2 mL/kg/hour for each kg between 10 and 20 kg, so 50 mL/hour. (PALS pg. 274)

9. Utilizing the 4-2-1 method, what is the hourly maintenance fluid for a 30-kg child?
   a. 50 mL/hour
   b. 60 mL/hour
   c. 70 mL/hour
   d. 80 mL/hour

   C – Maintenance fluid administration for children > 20 kg is 60 mL/hour + 1 mL/kg/hour for each kg > 20 kg, so 70 mL/hour. (PALS pg. 274)

10. What is the most common supply of water involved in submersion injury in children ages 1 to 4?
    a. Bathtub
    b. Pool
    c. Lake
    d. Ocean

    B – Submersion injury in children ages 1-4 occurs more in **pools**. Bathtubs are more common areas for submersion in infants. Encourage caregivers to supervise swimming and install pool barriers and alarms. Large bodies are water are common areas of submersion in adolescents, especially if there is a history of seizures or cardiac abnormalities such as prolonged QT interval.

11. What is the initial management of a child experiencing hives, facial swelling, and vomiting after eating a peanut butter cookie?
    a. Positive pressure ventilation
    b. Inhaled albuterol
    c. Intramuscular (IM) epinephrine
    d. Intravenous (IV) diphenhydramine

    C – IM epinephrine in the lateral thigh in the vastus lateralis muscle is the priority. (ENPC pgs. 103 and 166)

12. Flash capillary refill and bounding peripheral pulses are regularly assessed in which type of shock?
    a. Hyperdynamic septic shock
    b. Neurogenic shock from spinal cord injury
    c. Cardiogenic shock
    d. Obstructive shock

A – Flash capillary refill with warm, flushed skin and bounding peripheral pulses are seen in early **hyperdynamic septic shock**. (ENPC pgs. 103 and 150)

Professional Issues (12 Exam Questions, 10 Samples)

1. EMS brings in an unresponsive 15-year-old patient after an MVC. You are unable to reach his parents, so he is treated under which consent?
    a. Implied
    b. Express
    c. Involuntary
    d. Informed

A – **Implied consent allows treatment in an emergency** when the patient is unable to give consent. Express consent is an agreement to treat. Involuntary consent is utilized when an individual refuses consent for treatment, like suicidal patients. For informed consent, the patient must understand the risks and benefits. (ENPC pg. 21)

2. A 15-year-old female signs into the emergency department requesting treatment for vaginal discharge. Which of the following is **INCORRECT** about consent for minors?
    a. Emancipated minors may be allowed to provide consent regardless of age.
    b. Minors are frequently able to consent to treatment for pregnancy-related issues.
    c. Age of consent is 16-year-old in all US states.
    d. Minors are frequently able to consent to treatment for substance abuse or alcohol rehabilitation.

C – **Age of consent varies among state statutes**. Minors are frequently able to consent for treatment for STI's, addiction, and pregnancy. Emancipated minors may be allowed to consent regardless of age. (ENPC pg. 21)

3. A patient presents to the ED complaining of shortness of breath and states that he does not have insurance at the front desk. The patient is turned away from the ED because he states that he cannot afford to pay at the time of visit. What is the department in violation of?
    a. The Joint Commission
    b. EMTALA
    c. The CDC requirements
    d. The Center for Medicare and Medicaid Services Mandate (CMS)

B – EMTALA is a component of COBRA which states that a qualified provider must perform a medical screening exam and treatment to stabilize emergency medical conditions on all patients who present to the ED requesting emergency care. (ENPC pg. 25)

4. All the following are requirements of EMTALA (Emergency Medical Treatment And Labor Act), **EXCEPT**:
    a. Patients are stabilized to the extent possible by the referring facility prior to transfer.
    b. The provider does not need to secure an accepting physician if the patient is being transferred to a regional trauma center.
    c. Consent for transfer must be obtained from a patient or their representative after outlining risks of transport.
    d. A medical screening examination must be performed by a qualified medical provider regardless of the patient's ability to pay.

B - The sending provider must speak to the receiving provider and the patient **must be accepted** by the receiving facility prior to initiating transport. (ENPC pg. 25)

5. The following are true regarding forensic evidence collection, **EXCEPT**:
    a. Avoid cutting through stains and holes when cutting clothes off.
    b. Follow the proper chain of custody.
    c. Place evidence in plastic bags.
    d. The well-being of the patient should take precedence over forensic evidence collection.

   C – Forensic evidence should be placed in **paper bags**, not plastic. All the other options are correct (ENPC pg. 264)

6. Which ethnic group has the highest of childhood obesity in the United States (US)?
    a. White
    b. Black
    c. Hispanic
    d. Asian

   C – Hispanic ethnicity has the highest rate of childhood obesity in the US at 26.2 %, increasing their risk of hypertension and type 2 diabetes mellitus. Blacks have 24.8%, white 16.6%, Asian 9%. The risk of childhood obesity is 19.7% in the total US population.

7. Child-resistant packaging is which type of injury prevention?
    a. Primary
    b. Secondary
    c. Tertiary
    d. Qualitative

   A – The goal of primary injury prevention efforts is to avoid the injury. Examples include **child-resistant packaging**, safe playground materials, stair gates, and securing furniture and televisions.

8. Most water heaters default to what temperature?
    a. 120 degrees F (49 C)
    b. 130 degrees F (54 C)
    c. 140 degrees F (60 C)
    d. 150 degrees F (66)

   C – Most water heaters default at **140 degrees F** (60 C), advise caregivers to set no higher than 120 degrees F (49 C). A child's bath water temperature should be at 100 degrees F (38 C).

9. Discharge instructions for a pregnant patient should include taking which supplement to reduce the risk of neural tube defects?
    a. Iron
    b. Folic acid
    c. Vitamin D
    d. Calcium

   B – **Folic acid** prevents neural tube defects such as spina bifida by up to 70 percent.

10. EMTALA (Emergency Medical Treatment And Labor Act) is based on which nursing ethical principle?
    a. Beneficence
    b. Nonmaleficence
    c. Autonomy
    d. Justice

   D – EMTALA (Emergency Medical Treatment And Labor Act) is based on **social justice (fairness)** ensuring uninsured patients receive the same treatment as insured patients. (Sheehy pgs. 6 & 13)

1. Why is patient and family centered care (PFCC) important? (ENPC pg. 20)
2. What is the leading cause of death in children greater than 1 year of age? (ENPC pg. 21)
3. What type of consent is communicated verbally or written? (ENPC pg. 21)
4. What type of consent is used in an emergency? (ENPC pg. 21)
5. List some examples of potential allowances to minor consent? (ENPC pg. 21)
6. What are the components of the HEADS-ED Screening tool? (ENPC pgs. 22-23)
7. List some key components of effective discharge education? (ENPC pgs. 23-24)
8. Who is responsible for ensuring qualified transport personnel accompany the patient to a specialized pediatric center? (ENPC pg. 25)
9. Why is "one voice" an important communication consideration during a procedure? (ENPC pg. 33)
10. Why is it important to document the child's weight in kilograms (kgs)? (ENPC pgs. 33 and 60)
11. Why should you count an infant's respiratory rate for a full minute? (ENPC pg. 35)
12. What is the formula for remembering hypotension based on systolic blood pressure in children ages 1 to 10? (ENPC pgs. 34 and 99)
13. How do you measure preductal and post ductal saturation in a neonate suspected of having congenital heart disease? (ENPC pg. 35)
14. Why are rib fractures a red flag for child maltreatment? (ENPC pg. 36)
15. Why do you NOT wrap a tibial intraosseous needle circumferentially? (ENPC pg. 37)
16. What are the three components of the pediatric assessment triangle (PAT)? (ENPC. 49)
17. TICLS is a useful mnemonic for the assessment of general appearance. What is TICLS? (ENPC pgs. 49 and 77)
18. A child who is categorized as "P" or "U" utilizing the AVPU mnemonic to assess disability is triaged as which Emergency Severity Index (ESI) level? (ESI Triage 5th edition)
19. A 14-day-old with a temperature of 39 degrees Celsius (102.2 Fahrenheit) is categorized as which ESI Triage level? (ENPC 5th edition Chapter 6)
20. Patients who are post-ictal, suicidal, or suspected of having an ectopic pregnancy are triaged as which ESI level? (ESI Triage 5th edition)
21. Is Emergency Severity Index (ESI) triage acuity level ever downgraded? (ENPC pg. 57)
22. What is the correct order of vital sign assessment in pediatrics? (ENPC pg. 59)
23. Why do you listen to midaxillary breath sounds to confirm tracheal tube placement? (ENPC pg. 71)
24. Normal capillary refill is 2 seconds or less. Flash capillary refill (less than 1 second) is a sign of which shock state? (ENPC pgs. 72 and 103)
25. PERRL indicates pupils are equal, round, and reactive to light. How do you assess pupillary accommodation? (ENPC pg. 73)
26. In a pediatric patient with severe shock, how should you administer the 20 mL/kg fluid bolus? (ENPC pg. 73)
27. In hemorrhagic shock, what is the recommended volume of packed red blood cells and other blood products? (ENPC pgs. 72 and 164)
28. Why is it essential to insert a gastric tube immediately post endotracheal intubation? (ENPC pg. 76)
29. Which cranial nerves are assessed by tracking the patient's gaze through the six cardinal fields of extraocular movements? (ENPC pg. 78)
30. What is the first step of neonatal resuscitation? (ENPC. Pg. 84)
31. Which do you suction first in neonatal resuscitation, the mouth or nose? (ENPC. Pg. 84)
32. What is the single most important and effective step in neonatal resuscitation? (ENPC pg. 85)
33. What is the most common endocrine disease found in the neonate? (ENPC pg. 86)
34. What electrolyte disorder is seen when formula is diluted with excessive water? (ENPC pg. 86)
35. What medications used to reduce pain during procedures may cause methemoglobinemia? (ENPC pg. 87)
36. What is a complication of prostaglandin administration? (ENPC pg. 88)

37. What is the inborn error of metabolism where the body cannot break down phenylamine, an amino acid found in natural protein? (ENPC pg. 91)
38. What blood pressure change is seen in early shock? (ENPC pg. 98)
39. What is the most common type of shock seen in children? (ENPC pg. 101)
40. What are some causes of obstructive shock? (ENPC pg. 102)
41. What is pulsus paradoxus? (ENPC pg. 102)
42. What is the priority treatment for anaphylactic shock? (ENPC pg. 103)
43. What causes bradycardia and vasodilation in neurogenic shock? (ENPC pg. 103)
44. What are the most common symptoms of asthma? (ENPC pg. 121)
45. Why is ketamine the recommended agent for sedation prior to intubation of the patient experiencing an exacerbation of asthma? (ENPC pg. 122)
46. What are the hallmark symptoms of laryngotracheitis (LTB)? (ENPC pg. 124)
47. What isolation precautions are initiated in suspected pertussis "whooping cough?" (ENPC pg. 126)
48. Children secured with lap restraints only are at risk for what injuries? (ENPC pg. 131)
49. What burns are suspicious for child maltreatment? (ENPC pg. 133)
50. Why is a vented chest seal applied to an open chest wound instead of an occlusive dressing? (ENPC pg. 134)
51. How do you control external hemorrhage? (ENPC pg. 134)
52. What is the correlation between electrical injury and acute kidney injury? (ENPC pg. 136)
53. What is the American Burn Association formula for calculating fluid replacement in pediatric thermal burns? (ENPC pg. 137)
54. What medications are used to decrease intracranial pressure? (ENPC pg. 139)
55. What is a potential cause of petechiae above the nipple line? (ENPC pg. 150)
56. A diffuse erythematous rash with small papules that have a sandpaper texture are representative of what rash? (ENPC pgs. 154 and 201)
57. What medication is used to promote fluid administration in subcutaneous fluid therapy? (ENPC pg. 164)
58. Forceful, nonbilious vomiting after feeding with continual hunger is seen in what abdominal disorder typically seen in infants under 3 months of age? (ENPC pg. 167)
59. An air enema may be useful in which abdominal disorder characterized by intermittent abdominal pain and a sausage-shaped abdominal mass? (ENPC pgs. 167-169)
60. Which foods commonly trigger food protein-induced enterocolitis syndrome (FPIES)? (ENPC pg. 167)
61. Why are button batteries dangerous when ingested? (ENPC pgs. 178-179)
62. What reflex is generally absent in testicular torsion? (ENPC pgs. 184-185)
63. The rash of which communicable infection are described as "dewdrops on a rose petal"? (ENPC pg. 199)
64. A patient with varicella (chickenpox) is placed on which types of isolation? (ENPC pg. 199)
65. What are the hallmark signs and symptoms of measles? (ENPC pg. 200)
66. Blisters that scab with a characteristic "honey-colored" crust surrounding the nose and mouth are indicative of what contagious bacterial skin infection? (ENPC pg. 201)
67. What childhood rash is a common form of eczema? (ENPC pg. 202)
68. Nocturnal pruritis and burrows on the wrists, ankles, axillae, and around the waist are suggestive of what infestation? (ENPC pgs. 202-203)
69. Why is Flumazenil (Romazicon) no longer recommended in benzodiazepine overdose? (ENPC pg. 213)
70. What medications are used to treat tricyclic antidepressant (amitriptyline) overdoses? (ENPC pg. 217)
71. What medications are used to treat beta-blocker and calcium-channel blocker overdoses? (ENPC pg. 217)
72. What chelating agent is used in iron toxicity? (ENPC pg. 217-218)
73. Why is sodium bicarbonate utilized in salicylate overdose? (ENPC pg. 218)
74. Why is folic acid administered in methanol ingestion? (ENPC pg. 219)
75. Why is pulse oximetry unreliable in carbon monoxide poisoning? (ENPC pg. 221)
76. What is the treatment for carbon monoxide poisoning? (ENPC pg. 221)

77. What is the preferred antidote for cyanide poisoning? (ENPC pg. 221)
78. What is the initial management of the patient exposed to organophosphates? (ENPC pg. 222)
79. What are the antidotes for organophosphate (OP) exposure? (ENPC pgs. 222-223)
80. What is the first line agent to treat pediatric status epilepticus in a patient without IV access? (ENPC pg. 225)
81. What are signs/symptoms of hydrocephalus? (ENPC pgs. 231-232)
82. What is always the priority when caring for patients experiencing a violent outburst? (ENPC pg. 240)
83. How are extrapyramidal symptoms such as dystonia treated initially? (ENPC pg. 246)
84. What are characteristics of anorexia nervosa? (ENPC pg. 248)
85. What are characteristics of bulimia nervosa? (ENPC pg. 248)
86. What is the motivation for caregiver-fabricated illness (medical child abuse)? (ENPC pg. 256)
87. What mnemonic may be helpful to identify suspicious bruising? (ENPC pg. 257)
88. What are the hallmark findings in abusive head trauma? (ENPC pg. 259)
89. How is evidentiary forensic material stored? (ENPC pg. 264)
90. Why is asking "What happened to you?" better than asking "What is wrong with you?" (ENPC pg. 270)
91. What is "the pause?" (ENPC pg. 273)
92. Who are the experts when caring for a child with special healthcare needs? (ENPC pg. 280)
93. What medical disorders are seen in patients with Marfan's? (ENPC pg. 282)
94. What is the essential first step in caring for a patient with an insulin pump? (ENPC pg. 284)
95. What is the purpose of using "person-first" language? (ENPC pg. 286)
96. Hyperesthesia of the cheek and upper lip, periorbital edema, and diplopia are signs/symptoms of which ocular injury? (ENPC 5th edition pg. 184)
97. How do you treat a ruptured globe in the ED? (ENPC 5th edition pg. 187)
98. What is the treatment for orbital cellulitis? (ENPC 5th edition pg. 192)
99. What spider bite is initially painless but progresses into a "bullseye" necrotizing lesion? (ENPC 5th edition pg. 281)
100. What color does a colorimetric CO_2 detector turn in the presence of carbon dioxide? (Nellcor™ Adult/Pediatric Colorimetric CO2 Detector | Medtronic)

CPEN Critical Thinking Answers

1. Why is patient and family centered care (PFCC) important? PFCC improves patient outcomes, enhances the patient and family experience, heightens clinician and staff satisfaction, and better allocates resources.
2. What is the leading cause of death in children greater than 1 year of age? Injury is the leading cause of death.
3. What type of consent is communicated verbally or written? Expressed consent.
4. What type of consent is used in an emergency? Implied consent.
5. List some examples of potential allowances to minor consent? Mental health, prenatal care sexual health, and substance use.
6. What are the components of the HEADS-ED Screening tool? **H**ome, **E**ducation, **A**ctivities, **D**rugs/Alcohol, **S**uicidality, **E**motions, **D**ischarge.
7. List some key components of effective discharge education? Sit at eye level, use clear plain language in a nonjudgmental tone, consider using "Ask Me 3" or pictogram-based instruction sheets.
8. Who is responsible for ensuring qualified transport personnel accompany the patient to a specialized pediatric center? The transferring facility arranges appropriate transport of the unstable patient, in accordance with the provisions of EMTALA.
9. Why is "one voice" an important communication consideration during a procedure? One person talking lessens stimulation and helps create a nonthreatening environment.

10. Why is it important to document the child's weight in kilograms (kgs)? Pediatric medication dosing is based on kilograms, and double dosing may be lethal.
11. Why should you count an infant's respiratory rate for a full minute? Count for a full minute since an infant's breathing may be irregular with shorts periods of apnea.
12. What is the formula for remembering hypotension based on systolic blood pressure in children ages 1 to 10? The formula is < 70 + (2 x age in years) for children.
13. How do you measure preductal and post ductal saturation in a neonate suspected of having congenital heart disease? Measure pulse oximetry on the right hand and compare it to the measurement in either foot. If there is a difference in the two measurements by more than 3% or if either oxygen saturation is less than 90% there may be a heart defect.
14. Why are rib fractures a red flag for child maltreatment? Infant cartilage is bendable and more difficult to break.
15. Why do you NOT wrap a tibial intraosseous needle circumferentially? An early sign of IO infiltration is swelling behind the site, and it is easily missed if the site is covered.
16. What are the three components of the pediatric assessment triangle (PAT)? **A**ppearance, work of **B**reathing, and **C**irculation to the skin.
17. TICLS is a useful mnemonic for the assessment of general appearance. What is TICLS? **T**one, **I**nteractiveness, **C**onsolability, **L**ook, **S**peech.
18. A child who is categorized as "P" or "U" utilizing the AVPU mnemonic to assess disability is triaged as which Emergency Severity Index (ESI) level? A patient listed as "P" or "U" is triaged as ESI level 1.
19. A 14-day-old with a temperature of 39 degrees Celsius (102.2 Fahrenheit) is categorized as which ESI Triage level? One to 28-day-olds are assigned ESI level 2 if the temperature is > 38 degrees C (100.4 F)
20. Patients who are post-ictal, suicidal, or suspected of having an ectopic pregnancy are triaged as which ESI level? Level 2
21. Is Emergency Severity Index (ESI) triage acuity level ever downgraded? No, it is based on the patient's initial presentation.
22. What is the correct order of vital sign assessment in pediatrics? Respiratory rate, heart rate, blood pressure, then temperature assessment.
23. Why do you listen to midaxillary breath sounds to confirm tracheal tube placement? Referred breath sounds are common in a child's small chest.
24. Normal capillary refill is 2 seconds or less. Flash capillary refill (less than 1 second) is a sign of which shock state? Flash capillary refill and bounding pulses are a sign of warm hyperdynamic septic shock.
25. PERRL indicates pupils are equal, round, and reactive to light. How do you assess pupillary accommodation? Pupils constrict when focusing on an object near the nose after the patient looks at a distant object.
26. In a pediatric patient with severe shock, how should you administer the 20 mL/kg fluid bolus? Infuse the fluid bolus within 5 to 10 minutes using the pull-push method with a three-way stopcock.
27. In hemorrhagic shock, what is the recommended volume of packed red blood cells and other blood products? The recommended volume is 10 mL/kg per intravenous bolus.
28. Why is it essential to insert a gastric tube immediately post endotracheal intubation? Bag-mask ventilation causes gastric distension. Gastric distention may impair ventilation by impeding downward movement of the diaphragm. Gastric tube placement improves tidal volume.
29. Which cranial nerves are assessed by tracking the patient's gaze through the six cardinal fields of extraocular movements? Cranial nerves III, IV, and VI make your eyes do some tricks.
30. What is the first step of neonatal resuscitation? Warm, dry, and stimulate the neonate.
31. Which do you suction first in neonatal resuscitation, the mouth or nose? Use a bulb syringe to clear the mouth and then the nose.
32. What is the single most important and effective step in neonatal resuscitation? Positive-pressure ventilation.
33. What is the most common endocrine disease found in the neonate? Adrenal insufficiency from adrenal hyperplasia.

34. What electrolyte disorder is seen when formula is diluted with excessive water? Hyponatremia, which may induce seizures.
35. What medications used to reduce pain during procedures may cause methemoglobinemia? Lidocaine-based topical anesthetics like benzocaine may cause methemoglobinemia, a form of hemoglobin that does not carry oxygen, leading to cyanosis. Teething gels may also contain benzocaine. Treat methemoglobinemia with methylene blue.
36. What is a complication of prostaglandin administration? Apnea, so be prepared for possible endotracheal intubation. Caffeine may be administered as an antagonist to an apneic spell.
37. What is the inborn error of metabolism where the body cannot break down phenylamine, an amino acid found in natural protein? Phenylketonuria (PKU).
38. What blood pressure change is seen in early shock? Increased diastolic blood pressure leading to a narrowed pulse pressure.
39. What is the most common type of shock seen in children? Hypovolemic shock from vomiting, diarrhea, hemorrhage, and burns.
40. What are some causes of obstructive shock? Tension pneumothorax, cardiac tamponade, ductal-dependent lesions, hypertrophic cardiomyopathy, and massive pulmonary embolism.
41. What is pulsus paradoxus? A drop in blood pressure with inspiration.
42. What is the priority treatment for anaphylactic shock? Intramuscular (IM) epinephrine in the vastus lateralis.
43. What causes bradycardia and vasodilation in neurogenic shock? The damage from spinal cord injury above T6 results in disruption of sympathetic nervous system stimulation, leaving unopposed parasympathetic stimulation.
44. What are the most common symptoms of asthma? Wheezing and cough.
45. Why is ketamine the recommended agent for sedation prior to intubation of the patient experiencing an exacerbation of asthma? Ketamine is also a bronchodilator.
46. What are the hallmark symptoms of laryngotracheitis (LTB)? Inspiratory stridor and a barky cough.
47. What isolation precautions are initiated in suspected pertussis "whooping cough?" Initiate droplet precautions and report the highly contagious infection to public health officials.
48. Children secured with lap restraints only are at risk for what injuries? Lap restraint injuries include hollow organ injuries such as small bowel or stomach, and chance fractures of the lumbar spine.
49. What burns are suspicious for child maltreatment? Clearly demarcated burns of the lower legs to feet (sock-like), hands (scald gloves), or buttocks (doughnut pattern) due to intentional dunking in scalding water, or patterned burns from an iron or cigarette.
50. Why is a vented chest seal applied to an open chest wound instead of an occlusive dressing? To prevent air trapping.
51. How do you control external hemorrhage? Direct pressure, pressure dressing, wound packing, or tourniquets.
52. What is the correlation between electrical injury and acute kidney injury? Electrical injury causes muscle damage resulting in myoglobinuria and kidney damage.
53. What is the American Burn Association formula for calculating fluid replacement in pediatric thermal burns? The formula is 3 mL x kg x % TBSA burned. Half of the total is administered in the first 8 hours from the time the burn occurred, and the remaining half over the remaining 16 hours. Infuse to a goal urine output of 1-2 mL/kg/hour for infants, 1-1.5 mL/kg/hour for children, and .5 mL/kg/hour for adolescents. Monitor for myoglobinuria in electrical burns.
54. What medications are used to decrease intracranial pressure? Hypertonic saline and mannitol are used to reduce ICP. Avoid hypoxia and hypotension.
55. What is a potential cause of petechiae above the nipple line? Forceful vomiting or coughing.
56. A diffuse erythematous rash with small papules that have a sandpaper texture are representative of what rash? Scarlet fever.
57. What medication is used to promote fluid administration in subcutaneous fluid therapy? Hyaluronidase.

58. Forceful, nonbilious vomiting after feeding with continual hunger is seen in what abdominal disorder typically seen in infants under 3 months of age? Pyloric stenosis.
59. An air enema may be useful in which abdominal disorder characterized by intermittent abdominal pain and a sausage-shaped abdominal mass? Intussusception
60. Which foods commonly trigger food protein-induced enterocolitis syndrome (FPIES)? Milk, soy, rice, egg, or fish.
61. Why are button batteries dangerous when ingested? They emit electrical discharge, leak battery fluid that causes necrosis, erodes tissue, and may cause lead or mercury poisoning.
62. What reflex is generally absent in testicular torsion? The cremasteric reflex is the elevation of the testis when stroking the thigh.
63. The rash of which communicable infection are described as "dewdrops on a rose petal"? The crops of vesicles on the erythematous skin seen in chickenpox are sometimes described as "dewdrops."
64. A patient with varicella (chickenpox) is placed on which types of isolation? Standard, contact, and airborne isolation.
65. What are the hallmark signs and symptoms of measles? Measles (Rubeola) is distinguished by the 3 C's of cough, coryza, and conjunctivitis and Koplik spots on buccal mucosa. Infection control measures include standard and airborne precautions.
66. Blisters that scab with a characteristic "honey-colored" crust surrounding the nose and mouth are indicative of what contagious bacterial skin infection? Impetigo. Cleansing and moisturizing are important.
67. What childhood rash is a common form of eczema? Atopic dermatitis, treated with skin hydration.
68. Nocturnal pruritis and burrows on the wrists, ankles, axillae, and around the waist are suggestive of what infestation? Scabies, treat with topical permethrin cream.
69. Why is Flumazenil (Romazicon) no longer recommended in benzodiazepine overdose? Reversing the effects in benzodiazepine-dependent patients may result in seizures. And, if the patient has a seizure, benzodiazepines will be ineffective.
70. What medications are used to treat tricyclic antidepressant (amitriptyline) overdoses? Sodium bicarbonate, lipid emulsion, lidocaine, magnesium, and benzodiazepines.
71. What medications are used to treat beta-blocker and calcium-channel blocker overdoses? Glucagon, calcium, dextrose, and lipid emulsion.
72. What chelating agent is used in iron toxicity? Deferoxamine is the antidote for iron toxicity.
73. Why is sodium bicarbonate utilized in salicylate overdose? Sodium bicarbonate alkalinizes the urine increasing the elimination of salicylates and helps correct metabolic acidosis.
74. Why is folic acid administered in methanol ingestion? It may prevent retinal toxicity.
75. Why is pulse oximetry unreliable in carbon monoxide poisoning? Pulse oximeters cannot differentiate oxygenated hemoglobin from carboxyhemoglobin. Management of carbon monoxide poisoning is high-flow oxygen.
76. What is the treatment for carbon monoxide poisoning? High-flow oxygen
77. What is the preferred antidote for cyanide poisoning? Hydroxocobalamin
78. What is the initial management of the patient exposed to organophosphates? Decontamination by undressing the patient and washing with soap and water.
79. What are the antidotes for organophosphate (OP) exposure? Atropine and pralidoxime are the antidotes for OP exposure.
80. What is the first line agent to treat pediatric status epilepticus in a patient without IV access? Intramuscular or intranasal midazolam.
81. What are signs/symptoms of hydrocephalus? Irritability, high-pitched cry, increasing head circumference, bulging fontanelle, and sunset eyes.
82. What is always the priority when caring for patients experiencing a violent outburst? Staff safety is always the priority, and it may be best to remove yourself from the situation. Avoid being blocked from the exit.

83. How are extrapyramidal symptoms such as dystonia treated initially? Treat with diphenhydramine or benztropine (Cogentin).
84. What are characteristics of anorexia nervosa? A disproportionate fear of obesity, distorted body image, and refusal to eat.
85. What are characteristics of bulimia nervosa? Rapidly consuming large amounts of food followed by purging. Calloused hands, tooth erosion, esophageal erosion.
86. What is the motivation for caregiver-fabricated illness (medical child abuse)? Need for attention or to covertly manipulate or deceive authority figures.
87. What mnemonic may be helpful to identify suspicious bruising? The "TEN-4 FACES P" mnemonic refers to bruising of the torso, ear, or neck, frenulum, auricular, cheek, eyelid, subconjunctivae, and patterned injuries.
88. What are the hallmark findings in abusive head trauma? Subdural hemorrhage, retinal hemorrhage, skull fractures, and rib fractures.
89. How is evidentiary forensic material stored? Store forensic evidence in paper bags.
90. Why is asking "What happened to you?" better than asking "What is wrong with you?" It follows trauma-informed care approach avoiding retraumatization.
91. What is "the pause?" A period of silence after a patient's death to honor the life. It highlights the human aspect of healthcare, fostering staff well-being.
92. Who are the experts when caring for a child with special healthcare needs? The caregivers are the experts.
93. What medical disorders are seen in patients with Marfan's? Aortic dilation or aneurysms, mitral valve prolapse, and spontaneous pneumothorax.
94. What is the essential first step in caring for a patient with an insulin pump? Checking bedside glucose level.
95. What is the purpose of using "person-first" language? "Person-first" language is less stigmatizing and diminishes unconscious bias. "Special needs" may be considered condescending or patronizing.
96. Hyperesthesia of the cheek and upper lip, periorbital edema, and diplopia are signs/symptoms of which ocular injury? Orbital fracture.
97. How do you treat a ruptured globe in the ED? Do not instill eye drops and place a protective rigid shield over the affected eye.
98. What is the treatment for orbital cellulitis? Intravenous antibiotics and ophthalmology or otolaryngology consult.
99. What spider bite is initially painless but progresses into a "bullseye" necrotizing lesion? Brown recluse spider.
100. What color does a colorimetric CO_2 detector turn in the presence of carbon dioxide? Yellow indicates CO_2 presence in tracheal intubation.

1. Which type of consent is assigned when a legal guardian is not available, and the patient is incapable of giving permission for treatment? (ENPC pg. 21)
    a. Express
    b. Implied
    c. Informed
    d. Involuntary
2. You are the triage nurse assessing an unvaccinated child with fever, conjunctivitis, cough, a splotchy red rash of the face, and red specks with blue-white center on the buccal mucosa. Which is the priority? (ENPC pgs. 194 & 200)
    a. Place the patient immediately in a room with a closed door.
    b. Administer acetaminophen to treat fever.
    c. Prepare to assist with a lumbar puncture.
    d. Initiate IV access to administer antibiotics.
3. Which of the following responsibilities is **NOT** an EMTALA regulation? (ENPC pg. 25)
    a. Appropriate medical screening to determine if a medical emergency exists.
    b. Safe and medically necessary transfer of the unstable patient.
    c. Reporting of certain illnesses, injuries, and suspicions.
    d. Proper stabilization within the facilities capacity and capabilities.
4. Where is the preferred site to administer intramuscular (IM) injections in an infant?
    a. Dorsogluteal muscles of the buttock
    b. Vastus lateralis muscle of the thigh
    c. Deltoid muscle of the arm
    d. Ventrogluteal muscle of the hip
5. Which of the following statements regarding the pediatric assessment triangle (PAT) is **INCORRECT**? The PAT: (ENPC pg. 49)
    a. Utilizes visual, auditory, and tactile cues.
    b. Enables the nurse to quickly determine if the child is sick, sicker, or sickest.
    c. Consists of three components, appearance, work of breathing, and circulation to the skin.
    d. The TICLS mnemonic is useful in recalling what to look for when assessing appearance.
6. Utilizing the pediatric assessment triangle (PAT), a child who is lethargic and cyanotic is labeled as: (ENPC pgs. 48-65)
    a. Sick
    b. Sicker
    c. Sickest
    d. Expectant
7. A 21-day-old neonate with a temperature of 38.2 degrees Celsius (100.8 degrees Fahrenheit) would be assigned which Emergency Severity Index (ESI) level? (ENPC pgs. 54-55 and ESI Triage)
    a. ESI Level 1
    b. ESI Level 2
    c. ESI Level 3
    d. ESI Level 4
8. A child with ineffective airway clearance and respiratory distress due to anaphylaxis would be assigned which Emergency Severity Index (ESI) level? (ENPC pgs. 54-55 and ESI Triage)
    a. ESI Level 1
    b. ESI Level 2
    c. ESI Level 3
    d. ESI Level 4

9. Utilizing JumpSTART triage, a 5-year-old ambulatory child is assigned which tag color? (ENPC pgs. 58-60)
    a. Black
    b. Red
    c. Yellow
    d. Green
10. What is the correct order of emergency pediatric assessment? (pg. 59)
    a. Temperature, heart rate, respiratory rate, blood pressure.
    b. Heart rate, respiratory rate, blood pressure, temperature.
    c. Respiratory rate, heart rate, blood pressure, temperature.
    d. Temperature, respiratory rate, heart rate, blood pressure.
11. What is the appropriate initial fluid resuscitation for a child in hypotensive non-hemorrhagic hypovolemic shock? (ENPC pgs. 72 and 164 and PALS)
    a. 10 mL/kg of an isotonic solution over 5 to 10 minutes.
    b. 10 mL/kg of an isotonic solution over 20 to 60 minutes.
    c. 20 mL/kg of an isotonic solution over 5 to 10 minutes.
    d. 20 mL/kg of an isotonic solution over 20 to 60 minutes.
12. What are the initial steps in neonatal resuscitation? (ENPC pgs. 84-85 and NRP)
    a. Warm, dry, and stimulate the neonate.
    b. Initiate positive-pressure ventilation (PPV) at 40 to 60 breaths/minute.
    c. Initiate basic life support with three chest compressions to one breath.
    d. Administer epinephrine via umbilical catheter.
13. A drop in blood pressure with inspiration (pulsus paradoxus) is seen in which type of shock? (ENPC pg. 102)
    a. Hypovolemic
    b. Obstructive
    c. Cardiogenic
    d. Distributive
14. How do you achieve the "sniffing" position in the young child with a large occiput? (PALS pg. 148, ENPC pg. 71)
    a. Place padding beneath the child's shoulders and torso.
    b. Place the child in the ramped position at 30 degrees.
    c. Position the child on his left side in recovery position.
    d. Hyperextend the neck.
15. Which is INCORRECT regarding insertion of oropharyngeal airways (OPA) in pediatric patients? (PALS pg. 154, ENPC pg. 71)
    a. Measure from the corner of the mouth to the angle of the jaw.
    b. Rotate the oropharyngeal airway 180 degrees upon insertion.
    c. Utilize a tonsil-tip suction device to stabilize the tongue.
    d. Oropharyngeal airways are not indicated for use in pediatric patients.
16. A patient with which of the following conditions would require droplet isolation precautions? (ENPC pg. 126)
    a. Varicella (chickenpox)
    b. Scabies
    c. Impetigo
    d. Pertussis
17. Which of the following injuries is **NOT** commonly associated with "seat belt" sign? (ENPC pg. 131)
    a. Cervical spine fracture
    b. Lumbar chance fracture
    c. Small bowel injury
    d. Ruptured stomach

18. Prior to total body surface area (TBSA) calculation, what is the initial infusion rate of lactated ringers (LR) solution for a 10-year-old with a thermal burn? (ENPC pg. 137)
    a. 125 mL/hour
    b. 250 mL/hour
    c. 500 mL/hour
    d. 1000/mL/hour
19. Forceful nonbilious vomiting with persistent hunger is seen in which abdominal emergency? (ENPC pgs. 167-169)
    a. Appendicitis
    b. Pyloric stenosis
    c. Intussusception
    d. Volvulus
20. Which of the following is NOT a common complication of streptococcal pharyngitis? (ENPC pgs. 153-154)
    a. Glomerulonephritis
    b. Rheumatic fever
    c. Peritonsillar abscess
    d. Ludwig's angina
21. Koplik spots in the oral mucosa are the hallmark sign of which contagious viral illness? (ENPC pgs. 198-200)
    a. Rubeola (Measles)
    b. Hand, Foot, Mouth Disease
    c. Varicella (Chickenpox)
    d. Fifth Disease
22. A "slapped check" rash is the hallmark sign of which contagious viral illness? (ENPC pgs. 198-200)
    a. Rubeola (Measles)
    b. Hand, Foot, Mouth Disease
    c. Varicella (Chickenpox)
    d. Fifth Disease
23. A vesicular rash which appears as "dewdrops on a rose petal" is the hallmark sign of which contagious viral illness? (ENPC pgs. 198-200)
    a. Rubeola (Measles)
    b. Hand, Foot, Mouth Disease
    c. Varicella (Chickenpox)
    d. Fifth Disease
24. A pruritic rash on the palms and the soles, which worsens at night is the hallmark sign of which contagious skin infestation? (ENPC pgs. 198-204)
    a. Scabies
    b. Tinea Corporis (Ringworm)
    c. Lice
    d. Cimex lectularius (Bed Bugs)
25. A well-demarcated circular lesion with a hypopigmented center and a scaly raised edge is the hallmark sign of which contagious skin infestation? (ENPC pgs. 198-204)
    a. Scabies
    b. Tinea Corporis (Ringworm)
    c. Lice
    d. Cimex lectularius (Bed Bugs)
26. A pruritic rash in clusters of three or more is the hallmark sign of which skin infestation? (ENPC pgs. 198-204)
    a. Scabies
    b. Tinea Corporis (Ringworm)
    c. Lice
    d. Cimex lectularius (Bed Bugs)

27. N-Acetylcysteine is the antidote for which poisoning? (ENPC pgs. 213-214)
    a. Cardizem
    b. Acetaminophen
    c. Digoxin
    d. Elavil
28. Hydroxocobalamin is the antidote for which poisoning? (ENPC pgs. 213-214)
    a. Carbon monoxide
    b. Organophosphates
    c. Cyanide
    d. Ethylene glycol
29. Deferoxamine is the antidote for which poisoning? (ENPC pgs. 213-214)
    a. Cardizem
    b. Iron
    c. Labetalol
    d. Elavil
30. Ethanol oral or intravenous is the antidote for which poisoning? (ENPC pgs. 213-214)
    a. Ethylene glycol
    b. Acetaminophen
    c. Digoxin
    d. Elavil
31. A teenager who ingested some plants "to get high" is confused, bradycardic, and complains of yellow-green halos in his vision. The nurse suspects he ingested which plant? (Sheehy pgs. 407-408)
    a. Salvia
    b. Peyote
    c. Foxglove
    d. Morning glory
32. Which of the following medications is **NOT** indicated in the treatment of amitriptyline (Elavil) overdose? (ENPC pg. 217)
    a. Sodium bicarbonate
    b. Flumazenil
    c. Lidocaine
    d. Magnesium
33. What is the priority management of organophosphate toxicity? (ENPC pg. 222)
    a. Airway management
    b. Atropine
    c. Pralidoxime
    d. Decontamination
34. Overly diluted infant formula causes which dangerous electrolyte abnormality? (ENPC pgs. 227-228)
    a. Hypokalemia
    b. Hyperkalemia
    c. Hyponatremia
    d. Hypercalcemia
35. What does the "P" refer to in the "TEN-4 FACES P" mnemonic used to identify suspicious bruising in children? (ENPC pg. 257)
    a. Patterned injuries
    b. Purple
    c. Petechiae
    d. Purpura

36. Movement limitation, spasticity, and seizures are seen in which of the following disorders? (ENPC pgs. 281-282)
    a. Cerebral palsy
    b. Cystic fibrosis
    c. Down syndrome
    d. Marfan syndrome
37. Thick respiratory and gastrointestinal mucus is seen in which of the following disorders? (ENPC pgs. 281-282)
    a. Cerebral palsy
    b. Cystic fibrosis
    c. Down syndrome
    d. Marfan syndrome
38. Aortic aneurysms, spontaneous pneumothorax, and atlantoaxial subluxations are complications of which of the following disorders? (ENPC pgs. 281-282)
    a. Commotio cordis
    b. Cystic fibrosis
    c. Down syndrome
    d. Marfan syndrome
39. Intrathecal baclofen therapy is useful in the treatment of which disorder? (ENPC pg. 285)
    a. Cerebral palsy
    b. Cystic fibrosis
    c. Down syndrome
    d. Osteogenesis imperfecta
40. What is the first step of the pediatric nursing process? (ENPC Appendix A)
    a. Don personal protective equipment (PPE).
    b. Prepare the room.
    c. Activate the team and assign roles.
    d. Assess the pediatric assessment triangle (PAT).
41. Reye's syndrome is most common with the use of which medication?
    a. Aspirin
    b. Acetaminophen
    c. Ibuprofen
    d. Simethicone
42. Care of the infant with osteogenesis imperfecta includes: (ENPC pg. 282)
    a. Avoiding rectal temperatures.
    b. Lifting the patient under the neck and buttocks to change diaper.
    c. Inserting an intraosseous needle (IO) versus IV access.
    d. Applying a cervical collar to protect spine.
43. Which laboratory value is decreased in tumor lysis syndrome? (ENPC pg. 281)
    a. Uric acid
    b. Potassium
    c. Phosphorus
    d. Calcium
44. How many times would you fill a 20 mL syringe utilizing the pull-push technique for intravenous fluid resuscitation in a 5 kg infant? (ENPC pg. 73)
    a. Two
    b. Four
    c. Five
    d. Ten

45. Which is CORRECT regarding the care of a patient after a pit viper snake bite to the lower leg? (Sheehy pg. 368)
    a. Elevate the leg above the level of the heart.
    b. Apply an ice pack to the bite area.
    c. Apply a tourniquet or constricting band to the lower leg.
    d. Remove the shoe and monitor closely for edema.
46. What is the dose of rabies immunoglobulin injected into the wound after a raccoon bite? (Sheehy pg. 366)
    a. 10 IU/kg
    b. 20 IU/kg
    c. 30 IU/kg
    d. 50 IU/kg
47. What days is the rabies vaccine administered in pediatrics? (Sheehy pg. 366)
    a. Day 0 only
    b. Days 0 and 7
    c. Days 7 and 14
    d. Days 0, 3, 7, and 14
48. Hemophilia A is a coagulation disorder resulting from a congenital deficit of which clotting factor? (Sheehy pg. 389)
    a. Factor VIII
    b. Factor IX
    c. Factor XI
    d. Von Willebrand factor
49. Methotrexate may be administered in which obstetric emergency? (ENPC pg. 184)
    a. Ectopic pregnancy
    b. Placenta previa
    c. Abruptio placenta
    d. Pregnancy-induced hypertension
50. Which sign/symptom is seen more commonly in anorexia nervosa versus bulimia? (ENPC pg. 248)
    a. Calloused knuckles of fingers
    b. Eroded teeth
    c. Abnormally low body weight
    d. Broken blood vessels in eyes

CPEN Posttest Answers

1. **B** is the answer. Implied (emergency) consent is assigned when the legal guardian is not present, and the patient is incapable of giving permission for treatment. Expressed consent is communicated verbally or through written means.
2. **A** is the answer. Infection control measures for Rubeola (Measles) include standard and airborne precautions.
3. **C** is the answer. EMTALA requires a medical screening exam to determine if a medical emergency exists, stabilization within the facilities capabilities, and the transfer of unstable patients.
4. **B** is the answer. The vastus lateralis muscle of the anterolateral thigh is the preferred IM injection sire for infants. The deltoid muscle of the arm is used in adults for injections.
5. **A** is the answer. The pediatric assessment triangle (PAT) uses visual and auditory (not tactile) cues to obtain a quick general impression of the patient's physiologic status.
6. **C** is the answer. This child has an alteration of two or more of the three components of the PAT and is considered sickest.
7. **B** is the answer. Temperature > 38 degrees C (100.4 degrees F) is a neonate indicates a high-risk situation, ESI 2.
8. **A** is the answer. Any patient with ineffective airway clearance is assigned ESI level 1, requiring life-saving interventions.
9. **D** is the answer. If the child can walk, they are assigned to minor care (Green) to get a secondary triage utilizing the JumpSTART pediatric mass-casualty incident triage algorithm.
10. **C** is the answer. Start with the least invasive vital sign first, proceed to the most invasive last.
11. **C** is the answer. Administer 20 mL/kg isotonic crystalloid bolus over 5 to 10 minutes for hypotensive, non-hemorrhagic hypovolemic shock.
12. **A** is the answer. The initial steps in neonatal resuscitation are to warm, dry, and stimulate the neonate. Then open the airway and suction the mouth and then the nose.
13. **B** is the answer. Pulsus paradoxus (a drop in blood pressure with inspiration) is seen in obstructive shock due to increased intrathoracic pressure. Examples of obstructive shock are cardiac tamponade, tension pneumothorax, and ductal-dependent lesions.
14. **A** is the answer. Place the child supine and flex the neck forward at the shoulder level while extending the head. Place padding under the shoulders and upper torso of infants and under the occiput in children older than 2 years of age to prevent excessive flexion.
15. **B** is the answer. Gently insert the OPA directly into the oropharynx. The use of a tongue blade or tonsil-tip suction to depress the tongue be helpful. The rotation insertion technique for an oral airway is not recommended.
16. **D** is the answer. The child with suspected pertussis and their caregivers should be placed in isolation with standard and droplet precautions.
17. **A** is the answer. Injuries associated with "seat belt" sign include small bowel and stomach injury, chance fracture of the lumbar spine, and spleen and liver injuries.
18. **B** is the answer. The initial infusion rates of LR (prior to TBSA calculation) are 125 mL/hour for ages 5 and under, 250 mL/hour for ages 6-13, and 500 mL/hour for ages 14 and over. When TBSA is calculated, infuse 3 mL/kg/TBSA for children under 14 years of age with a thermal burn, 2 mL/kg/TBSA for ages 14 and over with a thermal burn, 4 mL/kg/TBSA for all ages electrical burn.
19. **B** is the answer. The classic presentation of pyloric stenosis is forceful, nonbilious vomiting after feeding, with persistent hunger. An olive-shaped mass may be palpated in the upper abdomen. Diagnosis is confirmed by ultrasound, and endoscopy may be required.
20. **D** is the answer. Untreated streptococcal infections can lead to the development of acute rheumatic fever, glomerulonephritis, and peritonsillar abscess.

21. **A** is the answer. The hallmark sign of rubeola (measles) is small grayish-blue Koplik spots in the oral mucosa. Initiate standard and airborne precautions for measles and contact public health authorities since it is highly contagious.
22. **D** is the answer. A "slapped cheek" rash is characteristic of Fifth disease from parvovirus B19, along with fever, runny nose, and a sore throat.
23. **C** is the answer. A vesicular rash which appears as "dewdrops on a rose petal" is characteristic of varicella (chickenpox). The patient requires standard, contact, and airborne isolation. Treatment includes topical calamine lotion to prevent scratching.
24. **A** is the answer. Scabies is a contagious parasitic skin infestation of mites that burrow into the skin, producing a pruritic rash which worsens at night. Wash linens in hot water and treat with topical permethrin.
25. **B** is the answer. Tinea corporis (ringworm) is a contagious fungal skin infection. Treat with a topical antifungal.
26. **D** is the answer. Cimex lectularius (bed bugs) bite exposed parts of the body such as arms, legs, feet, face, and neck in clusters of three or more bites. Wash linens in hot water, professional pest control may be required. Treatment includes antihistamines.
27. **B** is the answer. N-Acetylcholine (Acetadote) is the antidote for acetaminophen poisoning. A single dose of activated charcoal may be administered orally if the patient presents to the ED within an hour of ingestion. The initial dose of Acetadote is 150 mg/kg.
28. **C** is the answer. Hydroxocobalamin is the antidote for cyanide poisoning, metabolizing into vitamin B12. Cyanide prevents the tissues from extracting oxygen from the blood.
29. **B** is the answer. Deferoxamine (a chelating agent) is the antidote for iron poisoning, resulting in pink urine.
30. **A** is the answer. Ethanol and fomepizole are antidotes for methanol and ethylene glycol poisoning. Folic acid also enhances methanol elimination and reduces visual impairment.
31. **C** is the answer. Foxglove (digitalis purpurea) causes GI disturbances, bradycardia, and yellow-green halos in vision.
32. **B** is the answer. Tricyclic antidepressant (TCA) such as amitriptyline (Elavil) overdoses are treated with sodium bicarbonate, lipid emulsion, lidocaine, magnesium, and benzodiazepines.
33. **D** is the answer. Management of the patient with organophosphate exposure starts with decontamination by undressing and washing with soap and water. Antidotes include atropine (anticholinergic) and pralidoxime (nicotinic antidote).
34. **C** is the answer. Overly diluted formula may lead to hyponatremia and result in seizures.
35. **A** is the answer. The "TEN-4 FACES P" mnemonic is helpful for identifying suspicious bruising. The "P" refers to patterned injuries.
36. **A** is the answer. Cerebral palsy is a neuromuscular disorder characterized by limited movement and spasticity. Seizure activity is seen in 25-45% of children with cerebral palsy.
37. **B** is the answer. Cystic fibrosis is an autosomal recessive condition in which a defective gene alters the ability to regulate sodium and chloride channels in the body, resulting in mucoid thickening. Thick mucoid blocks airway clearance and digestion.
38. **D** is the answer. Marfan is an autosomal dominant trait that causes a connective tissue disorder. Patients are at risk for aortic dilation and aneurysm, mitral valve prolapse, atlantoaxial subluxation, and spontaneous pneumothorax.
39. **A** is the answer. Intrathecal baclofen therapy is used to decrease spasticity in patients with cerebral palsy. Baclofen withdrawal may cause seizures and hyperthermia.
40. **C** is the answer. The first step of the pediatric nursing process is to activate the team and assign roles, like "pit crew" CPR taught in PALS. Then prepare the room and don personal protective equipment.
41. **A** is the answer. Children recovering from a viral infection such as chicken pox or flu are most at risk for Reye's syndrome, especially if treated with aspirin. High ammonia levels are seen in Reye's syndrome.

42. **B** is the answer. Slide your hand under the buttock to lift the infant with osteogenesis imperfects, do not lift the baby by the ankles or legs.
43. **D** is the answer. Tumor lysis syndrome results in hyperuricemia, hyperkalemia, hyperphosphatemia, and hypocalcemia.
44. **C** is the answer. Fluid boluses are 20 mL/kg, so fill the 20 mL syringe 5 times for a 5-kg infant.
45. **D** is the answer. Remove potentially constrictive clothing immediately. Do not apply ice or a tourniquet to the bite. Position the extremity at the level of the heart to decrease the chance of compartment syndrome.
46. **B** is the answer. 20 IU/kg is the dose of Rabies Immunoglobulin (HRIG) for all ages. Infiltrate it into the wound or administer intramuscular. 60,000 persons receive PEP, only 1-3 cases of rabies in the US.
47. **D** is the answer. Administer the rabies vaccine on days 0, 3, 7, and 14. Vaccines are administered in the vastus lateralis muscles in infants.
48. **A** is the answer. Hemophilia A is a congenital deficit of Factor VIII, which is included in cryoprecipitate.
49. **A** is the answer. Methotrexate may be administered to end a pregnancy.
50. **C** is the answer. Anorexia is characterized by abnormally low body weights and an intense fear of gaining weight. Bulimia is characterized by calloused knuckles, eroded teeth, and broken blood vessels in eyes due to excessive vomiting.

Made in United States
North Haven, CT
02 September 2026

17828174R00043